WHOLENESS
OR TRANSCENDENCE?

ALSO BY GEORG FEUERSTEIN

(Selections)

Sacred Paths
Holy Madness
The Encyclopedic Dictionary of Yoga
Yoga: The Technology of Ecstasy
The Yoga Sutra: A New Translation and Commentary
Introduction to the Bhagavad-Gita
Sacred Sexuality
Structures of Consciousness
Jean Gebser: What Color Is Your Consciousness?

WHOLENESS
OR TRANSCENDENCE?

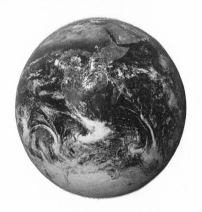

ANCIENT LESSONS
FOR THE EMERGING
GLOBAL CIVILIZATION

GEORG FEUERSTEIN

PUBLISHED FOR THE
PAUL BRUNTON PHILOSOPHIC FOUNDATION BY
LARSON PUBLICATIONS

International Standard Book Number: 0-943914-58-2
Library of Congress Catalog Card Number: 92-60590

Manufactured in the United States of America

Published for the
Paul Brunton Philosophic Foundation
by Larson Publications
4936 State Route 414
Burdett, New York 14818 USA

99 97 96 95 94 93 92

10 9 8 7 6 5 4 3 2 1

Book and cover design/production: Paperwork, Ithaca, New York

CONTENTS

ACKNOWLEDGEMENTS

 I AM GREATLY INDEBTED to several friends and colleagues. For the original version, written in 1973, I had the invaluable stylistic assistance of my friend Caroline Phillips, Ph.D. Franceska Freemantle, Ph.D., kindly read through some of the later chapters, making a number of helpful suggestions. For the present version, I owe thanks to ever-helpful John White; to my friend Claudia Bourbeau, who happily and deftly entered the bulk of the manuscript on computer; to my friend and neighbor Loretta Higgins, whose always timely body-work ensured my physical well-being; to my wife, Trisha, who applied her critical pencil to the printout and whose love nourished my inner being; to my splendid editor, Paul Cash, who is a Taoist in the art of editing; to Colin Wilson, who, across the Atlantic Ocean, kindly carved out time from his busy schedule to provide this book with a foreword, and not least to Larson Publications for adopting this work and publishing it so swiftly.

FOREWORD

BY COLIN WILSON

 I OWE A considerable debt of gratitude to Georg Feuerstein for drawing my attention to the work of Jean Gebser, who seems to me possibly the most important thinker of the twentieth century; this foreword is an attempt to repay a small part of that debt.

And what has a modern European philosopher—who once commented that "Yoga techniques appropriate to the Orient are most likely not in accord with our consciousness structure"—to do with a book devoted to Yoga and Oriental philosophy? To answer that, I must attempt my own brief exposition of Gebser's basic ideas.

Gebser argues that the discovery of perspective by Renaissance artists was a major evolutionary step in the history of the human race. In the second chapter of his masterpiece, *The Ever-Present Origin*, Gebser quotes at length that amazing letter written by Petrarch in which the poet describes climbing Mount Ventoux, between the Alps and the Cevennes. Petrarch is known to history as the first man who climbed a mountain simply to see the view from the top. And what he saw from Mount Ventoux was a revelation *of space*, of vast horizons. It was as if his consciousness had left his brain and floated out like a bird over the mountains. And contemporary artists were making the same discovery of space; through perspective they learned to create the same illusion of space on a flat plane.

Now Gebser argues that before this date, human consciousness was "unperspectival" (I prefer to translate it "non-perspectival"). Egyptian art is "flat," and so was Egyptian consciousness. We use the phrase "to put something in perspective" to mean to rise above our narrow personal viewpoint. Zola's peasants are still living in a state of non-perspectival consciousness, trapped in their petty ego-consciousness. Even Dante, Petrarch's great contemporary, seems trapped in a narrow and rather malicious viewpoint, so the *Commedia* has more than a touch of paranoia. But Petrarch taught human consciousness to "open up" and fly like a bird.

The "perspectival age" continued down to our own time. But now, says Gebser, human consciousness is entering a new phase of "aperspectival consciousness," a consciousness that is not confined to a single viewpoint but can move as freely as the consciousness of a god. When I read Gebser's description of aperspectival consciousness, I knew instantly what he meant.

When I was sixteen, I left school and had to take a job in a factory. It depressed me intensely. So when I came home, I used to retire to my bedroom and read poetry for hours—everything from Spenser and Milton to Yeats and Eliot. Gradually, the depression would lift, like a weight being raised, and at the end of an hour or so, I would experience a curious sensation of freedom—the *ability to embrace opposites*, like a monkey able to swing from branch to branch on either side of a tree, or even leap across a gap to another tree. This swinging from "branch to branch"—i.e., from Shakespeare to Poe, from Dante to Whitman, from Chaucer to Auden—was, I suggest, what Gebser means by aperspectival consciousness.

To put it crudely, you might say that non-perspectival consciousness could be compared to a straight line, possessing only one dimension; perspectival consciousness has an extra dimension, like a square. Aperspectival consciousness would possess yet another dimension, like a cube.

Gebser also speaks of what he calls "integral consciousness," which is defined by Feuerstein thus:

> The intensified consciousness of which Gebser speaks is . . . a consciousness that does not seek escape from the present. It is founded on the acceptance of the present, without being fixated on the present or confined by the constraints of the past, and without being either fearful of, or insensitive to, the future. This intensified consciousness is, therefore, not compressed into the molds of the rational consciousness. It is indeed not exhausted by any of the structures that constitute our total psychomental environment. It tran-

scends all the mind forms or molds created in the course of our evolution as conscious beings. It transcends them but it does not exclude them.

As an example of integral consciousness, I like to cite that scene in *From Here to Eternity* where Prewett is sitting in the PX drinking beer. He has no reason to feel happy: because the army is trying to force him to box, and because he is determined not to box, his superiors are giving him hell. Yet he is suddenly overwhelmed with a wonderful sense of sheer happiness, and thinks: "My God, I love the army . . ." For me, this is the essence of integral consciousness—that total affirmation.

Now in his book *Structures of Consciousness*, which is a study of Gebser's work, Feuerstein quotes Mircea Eliade to the effect that one of India's greatest discoveries is "the idea of consciousness as witness, of consciousness freed from its psychophysical structures and their temporal conditions." And in the Introduction to the present book, he speaks of the two basic spiritual orientations: the transcendent, "the quest for the eternal, beyond body, mind, and world," and the holistic, which "respects the fact that we live in a material universe with its own peculiar demands" and "favors the cultivation of spiritual experiences *and their integration with everyday existence*" (my italics).

This must be seen as the central theme of this important book, and as the answer to the objection that was my own first reaction to the typescript of *Wholeness or Transcendence?*—"Who needs another book about Eastern philosophy?" This may look like a book on Yoga and Buddhism, but its perspective is essentially that of Gebser, and its originality lies in its Gebserian approach, which looks upon India's civilization—its spirituality, notably Yoga—as a particular form of consciousness.

Widespread interest in Eastern religion began with the publication of Sir Edwin Arnold's *Light of Asia*, a poem on the life of the Buddha, published in 1879. In 1929, L. Adams Beck did for Eastern philosophy what Will Durant had done for European philosophy, and *The Story of Oriental Philosophy* achieved a well-deserved popularity. But it was the "transcendental" aspect of Oriental philosophy that appealed to Western intellectuals who felt deprived of their own religious tradition. They liked the assertion that this world is *maya*, or illusion, and that man should turn his back on *maya* to contemplate the eternal reality of *brahman*, whose essence is identical with that of the individual soul.

Buddhism also springs out of this attitude of "turning away"; the legend tells how the child Gautama, protected by his parents from all knowledge of misery, saw first an old man, then a sick man, then a dead man, and sought the path of enlightenment as an escape from the misery of human existence.

I fell under the spell of the *Bhagavad-Gita* at the age of sixteen, at the time I was working in the factory and fighting off depression: It had the effect of enabling me to gain control of my own mind. The *Dhamma-Pada*, the basic Buddhist text, was equally important to me. Yet having escaped the emotional tempests of adolescence, I began to feel that life was not quite as bad as the Buddha had painted it, and that there was also a great deal to be said for the more cheerful vision of Rabelais. My old friend Arthur Guirdham, the author of many books on reincarnation, is convinced that he was a Cathar in a previous existence, and wholeheartedly embraces the Manichean belief that matter is evil and spirit is good. When we argue about this, I point out to him that, according to the Book of Genesis, God looked on his handiwork "and saw that it was good."

It was in a book called *The Occult*, written twenty years ago, that I coined the term "Faculty X," which is basically what Gebser meant by integral consciousness. The simplest example of Faculty X can be found in the passage in *Swann's Way*, in which Proust describes how, tasting a cake dipped in herb tea, he experienced an exquisite sense of pleasure. "I had ceased to feel mediocre, accidental, mortal." Then he realizes that the taste of the madeleine has brought back, with total reality, his childhood in a little village called Combray. Such moments reveal that, in some sense, time is an illusion. But Proust's "Faculty X" was switched on quite accidentally, without any yogic discipline. It is what G.K. Chesterton once called "absurd good news," and is closely related to what Abraham Maslow called "peak experience."

It seems to me that this experience offers a new solution to the problem that the Buddha solved by world rejection. Our most basic human tendency is to feel "defeated" by what Heidegger called "the triviality of everydayness." Some of the most fashionable modern writers, from Gottfried Benn to Samuel Beckett, are convinced that life is a tale told by an idiot, a long drawn out defeat. Georg Feuerstein feels that this is one of the most dangerous drawbacks of mere "rational consciousness," a deficient and neurotic form of consciousness.

Nietzsche was the first to raise the possibility of a wholly unneurotic kind of consciousness, Zarathustra's total affirmation. Rilke symbolized the same notion in "The Angels" and in "Orpheus"—the notion of *dennoch preisen*, to "praise in spite of." And here we are getting very close to Gebser's integral consciousness. The basic notion here is of a deep internal certainty that life is good, that objective meaning really exists. If we can feel this total *intellectual* certainty, then the nagging romantic hunger to *feel and see* "the answer" suddenly appears to be a kind of self-indulgence. A deprived child may cling to anyone who offers him affection; an emotionally satisfied child has no need for constant reassurance.

At this point in human evolution, there appears for the first time the possibility of a human being who is as basically unaffected by problems as an ocean liner is by heavy seas. He *is* affected, of course—so is the liner—but there is not the slightest possibility of being sunk by them. Total *intellectual* certainty will replace the need for Arjuna's vision of God or the ecstasies of the Romantics. As to the grim stoicism of existential thinkers like Camus, Sartre, and Heidegger, it will be dismissed as an example of Feuerstein's "rational consciousness"—which, as he remarks, is an evolutionary cul-de-sac.

And who is Georg Feuerstein? A magazine interview he sent me contained at least the basic answers to that question. Born in 1947 into a Lutheran family, he found himself rejecting their beliefs—or rather, the fact that they did not take them seriously enough. This is the standard complaint of all men born with a powerful religious urge, and I presented a gallery of them in my second book *Religion and the Rebel*—Boehme, Pascal, Kierkegaard, Newman.

As a teenager Feuerstein came upon Paul Brunton's *In Search of Secret India*, which is heady stuff for anyone looking for belief. Brunton's book opens with an account of an interview with an Egyptian "magician" who was able not only to read his mind, but also to somehow write the answers to his questions on a folded sheet of paper that Brunton was holding his hand. In reply to Brunton's question as to how he did it, Mahmoud Bey replied—as ninety-nine percent of true "magicians" would—through spirits. I imagine that most modern readers—even of books on Yoga—would dismiss such an idea as nonsense. So would I twenty years ago; now I accept it.

Paul Brunton was for Feuerstein what Madame Blavatsky was for the poet Yeats. In the magazine interview, he comments: "The notion of withdrawing into oneself, ascending along the spinal column to illuminate the psychic center in the brain, and then forgetting about the world, escaping the cosmos, appealed to me." Feuerstein adds: "I was not allowed to be a yogi in a cave. Everything conspired to draw me back into life." And his friendship with Jean Gebser during the last years of the philosopher's life brought a new and powerful cultural orientation. It was the revelation of Gebser that led him to write *Wholeness or Transcendence?* from a Gebserian standpoint. This is most clearly presented in this book's final pages, where Feuerstein speaks of *sahaja-yoga*, a basic acceptance of reality, which is obviously the reverse of the "world rejection" of the Manichees and Cathars.

Feuerstein and I have followed parallel paths. My own starting point was the Romanticism of Goethe, Schiller, and Novalis, with its sense that there *is* a far more intense, ecstatic way to live, and the subsequent collapse of that romantic dream into life-failure and despair. In *Zarathustra*, Nietzsche recognized that the answer to the problem lies in strength, in "great health." Nietzsche himself never saw the "promised land," partly because of illness, partly because he was never able to devise a *discipline* that would enable him to achieve his objective. Feuerstein has always recognized instinctively that the answer lies in a discipline, and the present book is almost a record of his own quest.

Shaw remarked in *Man and Superman*: "The artist's work is to show us ourselves as we really are. Our minds are nothing but this knowledge of ourselves; and he who adds a jot to such knowledge creates new mind as surely as any woman creates new men." In Shaw's sense, Georg Feuerstein is a creator of new mind, and deserves to be regarded as an artist as much as a philosopher.

INTRODUCTION

THE GLOBAL CONTENT

 Contemporary life is replete with global problems and global opportunities, and we are undoubtedly on the threshold of a new world. What is unclear is whether that world will be fit for human life.

Dour skeptics prognosticate, in Spenglerian vein, the end of human civilization. Religious fundamentalists interpret this gloom-and-doom event as the Lord's final reckoning, which will be followed by the resurrection of the faithful and the eternal condemnation of unbelievers.

In contrast, naive "New Age" enthusiasts blithely affirm the dawning of a new golden era, ignoring the countless problems bedeviling our troubled planet. The New Age vision of a world free from war, destructive competitiveness, and intolerance is healthy, even if idealistic. Yet, hopefulness and positive thinking alone are not enough to usher in the longed-for new world. Genuine personal change combined with wise and efficient social action is essential.

We certainly need such positive ideals. However, we must not romanticize the possibilities inherent in our present situation. We must be realistic. As realists, we will appreciate the enormous difficulties confronting us, individually and collectively. Sustained by our lofty idealism, but without naïveté, we can then actively search for optimal pathways through the present civilizational maze.

What is certain is that our quest will succeed only to the degree that our thinking, planning, and acting are global. The well-known futurist Willis Harman has spoken of the need for a "global mind change," amounting to a new Copernican revolution.[1] To be sure, there are no parochial solutions to the contemporary crisis.

We cannot even be whole as individuals without taking the larger context fully into account. This becomes clear when we consider the issue of health. We must not expect full personal health so long as our environment is polluted. Without physical well-being, however, we are hard-pressed to maintain our psychological balance, or inner harmony. Without such harmony, it is difficult to think and act in wise measure.

The time has come when we are no longer able to disown any part of ourselves, our species, or our planet. We are one being. To preserve this grand vision in all our actions is the formidable challenge before us today.

THE EAST/WEST DIALOGUE

As many eminent thinkers have pointed out, in our endeavor to meet the exigencies of our era, we would do well to draw from the combined experience of all of humanity, especially the Eastern branch of the human family. It was the Orient, after all, that served as the cradle of human civilization—Sumer, Egypt, India, and China. Hence we can expect to find in those cultures the precious distillate of several millennia's worth of lessons.

There are those who maintain that the dialogue between East and West is "old hat," claiming that it has in any case been scarcely fruitful. Evoking the famous line from Kipling that "East is East and West is West, and never the twain shall meet," they argue that we must now get on with the business of our Western civilization. I believe this view to be sadly mistaken, shortsighted, and damaging. Besides, the next line in Kipling's "The Ballad of East and West" significantly reads: "But there is no East and West." In other words, the world is one.

It is true that the labels "East" and "West" are imprecise and subject to misapplication. But so are many other labels that we frequently use, such as "reality," "consciousness," "love," "progress," and "duty." Human language is inherently elastic, and we are constantly negotiating the pitfalls of this ambiguity. "East" and "West" are shorthand expressions for rather complex historical realities, and as long as we remain sensitive to this fact we can avoid misusing these labels.

Some critics argue that we should now cultivate the South/

North dialogue, the "South" being especially Latin America and Africa. This is of course to the point. But we should not abandon the East/West dialogue in the process. Rather, we need to broaden our base to include also the South/North axis. We need a global dialogue, in which the East/West discourse holds a place of special importance.

It is special because our Western civilization, which increasingly dominates the entire planet, has largely been built on the foundations of Eastern cultures. *Ex oriente lux.* Despite its rampant secularization, our Western civilization is in many respects still Christian. And Christianity of course started as a small Middle-Eastern sect within Judaism, subsequently coming under the influence of various Eastern traditions through the mediation of Gnosticism and Neoplatonism.

Moreover, despite several decades of dialogue between East and West, we have by no means fully understood the potential contribution of the Eastern half of humanity. This is particularly true of the vast civilization that was born in India over five thousand years ago. More than any other civilization, it has excelled in understanding the subtle modulations of the human mind. This is amply shown in the world's most refined psychotechnology, which widely goes by the name of Yoga but which is far more comprehensive than it is generally thought to be in the West.

To put it differently, India is a unique repository for what has been called the "perennial philosophy." This term comprises the great spiritual traditions, which attempt to furnish viable answers to the great existential questions that sooner or later every thoughtful individual must ask: Who am I? Whence do I come? Whither do I go? What must I do?

The present book is an effort to understand the Indian civilization from an evolutionary perspective that is meaningful to our contemporary global situation and our quest for transcendence and wholeness.

GLOBAL MIND CHANGE AND THE INTEGRAL CONSCIOUSNESS

There are many ways of approaching the global dialogue. An evolutionary perspective naturally commends itself. In this work I

avail myself, specifically, of the evolutionary model elaborated by
the Swiss cultural historian Jean Gebser.[2] This model is based on
the idea that human consciousness has undergone a series of trans-
mutations, leading from archaic humanity to modern *Homo sapiens
sapiens*.

Gebser speaks of structures of consciousness, which are distinct styles of perceiving and understanding the world. He distinguishes, in chronological order, four such major configurations:

1. *Archaic consciousness*, which is dominated by instinct and
characterized by the identity between subject and object. We
may surmise that this type of consciousness was present in
Homo habilis and perhaps still earlier hominids. It is the type
of consciousness present in the newborn baby.

2. *Magical consciousness*, which may have emerged with Homo
erectus or the Neanderthals, operates with only a rudimentary
self-sense. This is a visceral consciousness, marked by strong
emotionality. This consciousness is typical of the young child.

3. *Mythic consciousness*, which was probably typical of the Cro-
Magnons, is associated with the fully lateralized brain, language, and imaginative ability. It operates on the basis of
polarity rather than duality, and its symbol is the circle. The
identity is still defined by the "we" of the group rather than by
the "I" of the crystallized ego.

4. *Mental consciousness*, which fully crystallized during the
"axial period," the era of the Buddha, Lao Tzu, Pythagoras,
and Socrates. It is a strictly dualistic "either/or" consciousness, with a strong individualistic sense of identity (the
"ego"), which is epitomized in Protagoras' maxim that "Man
is the measure of all things." During the past several centuries,
this consciousness has congealed into the "rational" consciousness, which is fatally imbalanced.

   It is important to understand the difference between the mental consciousness and its deficient, rational mode. For Gebser, the
"rational" consciousness is not merely sober, logical thinking but
rather a whole way of looking at life through reductionistic
glasses. It is a consciousness that, unlike the mental consciousness

characteristic of much of classic Greek thought, lacks intrinsic balance. It is associated with an inflated self-sense and epitomized in the philosophy of extreme individualism, which decries altruism. The rational consciousness is the matrix of scientific materialism, virulent ethnocentrism, terrorism, and existential neuroses. It is a deficient form of consciousness, giving birth to deficient social and cultural manifestations. Far from being the summit of human accomplishment, the rational consciousness is an evolutionary cul-de-sac.

Luckily, life is an inexhaustible reservoir of possibilities and always contains the seeds of transformation. Thus, already in the 1950s, Gebser detected an emerging fifth structure of consciousness, which he called "integral." This corresponds roughly to Willis Harman's "new paradigm," Duane Elgin's "integral awareness," Peter Russell's "global brain," Charles Reich's "Consciousness III," and Marilyn Ferguson's "Aquarian Conspiracy."[3] Gebser carefully delineated the properties of the integral structure of consciousness, and from his descriptions we gather the following basic characteristics.

The integral consciousness is associated with ego-transcendence (rather than egolessness), self-transparency, freedom from anxiety (especially from the fear of time), openness, emotional availability and fluency, participatory freedom, personal responsiveness, bodily presence (rather than abstraction from life), the ability for genuine intimacy, equanimity, reverence for all life, the capacity for service, and love.

Gebser called the integral consciousness a mutation. However, unlike biological mutations, which proceed autonomously toward ever greater specialization, the mutation of the integral consciousness demands our conscious collaboration in order to become fully effective. We must submit to the difficult task of personally actualizing the essential features of the integral consciousness, such as self-knowledge, global thinking, and social responsibility.

Without this personal actualization of integral values, it will not be possible to replace the deteriorated mental-rational consciousness that has led to today's global crisis. Consequently, humanity's future would be more than uncertain.

TWO FUNDAMENTAL SPIRITUAL ORIENTATIONS

We cannot truly gauge the significance of the present without understanding the past, for the past is still present in us. The diverse structures of consciousness are not merely evolutionary stages in humanity's march through time, but they are the very building blocks of our psyche. Therefore we can better understand who we are by seeking to understand the developmental history of human consciousness.

The primary object of this book, then, is to trace and delineate the fundamental criteria that underlie the evolution of India's spiritual heritage as expressive of particular modes of consciousness. More specifically, I aim to show that India's spirituality embraces two great overarching orientations, or tendencies, which must be strictly distinguished. One orientation pertains to the mythic structure of consciousness; the other shows distinct integrative or holistic characteristics.

These two cognitive-cultural vectors have coexisted and complemented one another for countless generations in the long history of Indian civilization. Together they are responsible for the unimaginable wealth of experiential and philosophical knowledge that India holds in store for the unbiased student.

The first orientation is best expressed in the ideal of *transcendence*, the quest for the eternal beyond body, mind, and world. It is the "up and out" attitude of the ascending consciousness that views life as pain and suffering and endeavors to exit from the finite realm to merge with the blissful infinite.

This vertical orientation defines itself against the sharply contrasting attitude of the common person who behaves as if the limited material realm is all there is to reality. This horizontal, "flat" orientation to life recognizes no higher dimension but is thoroughly materialistic, exhausting itself in the pursuit of ephemeral goals.

In contrast to the vertical (transcendentalist) and the horizontal orientation, the *holistic* tendency seeks to preserve the integrity of life. It respects the fact that we live in a material universe with its own peculiar demands, and it fully takes into account that life is a mystery extending immeasurably beyond the material realm into the spiritual dimension. Therefore, without denying the body and the world, the holistic orientation favors the cultivation of spiritual experiences and their integration with everyday existence. This is the broad framework in which the present book needs to be placed. It is not so much addressed to specialists, though they too may find some new material, but is rather intended to serve the growing community of those who seek to learn from the experience of Eastern humanity.

ABOUT THIS BOOK

This book offers a cross-sectional view of the entire complex of Indian spirituality, with special reference to the omnipresent and ramifying tradition of Yoga.

Part One deals with the *mythic* variant of spirituality, that is, those schools that espouse transcendence as their primary goal. Here I have taken as my principal model the eightfold path of Classical Yoga, with complementary side-glances at Vedanta, Buddhism, Jainism, and other liberation teachings that contain a strong mythic component.

Part Two examines those tendencies within India's spirituality that can be said to be *integral* or *holistic*. These are highlighted in the examples of the teaching of the famous *Bhagavad-Gita* ("Lord's Song"), Mahayana Buddhism, Tantrism, and Hatha-Yoga.

I was obliged to confine the material rigorously to a representative selection, and the treatment had to remain skeletal. I have dealt with some of these themes in more detail elsewhere, notably in my books *Yoga: The Technology of Ecstasy* (1989) and *Holy Madness* (1991).

Wherever possible I have let the Indian sages and thinkers voice their own opinions. My translations from the Sanskrit are as literal as possible, and all interpretative matter, added to make the generally rather elliptic Sanskrit texts intelligible, is enclosed in square brackets.

Seventeen years have past since the publication of the original version of this book, which was titled *The Essence of Yoga*. In the interim, my understanding and appreciation of the astounding complexities of India's spiritual heritage have deepened considerably, and I have come to see a number of things more clearly. This is reflected in the extensive changes made in preparing the present enlarged edition.

This volume complements my book *Structures of Consciousness* (1987), an introduction to the ideas of Jean Gebser which are applied here to the great cultural configurations of Indian humanity. The present undertaking is a practical exercise in demonstrating the usefulness of the Gebserian model.

I see all my works as constituting a symphony that is being created even as my own life unravels itself. The insights I have gained from my studies of India's spirituality, with its extensive psychotechnology, have greatly informed my personal life and spiritual practice. In communicating them, I embody the hope that they can also be useful to others who, like me, are trying to find their bearings in our compassless postmodern civilization.

GEORG FEUERSTEIN
Summer 1992

NOTES

1. See W. Harman, *Global Mind Change: The Promise of the Last Years of the Twentieth Century* (Indianapolis, IN: Knowledge Systems, 1988).

2. See J. Gebser, *The Ever-Present Origin* (Athens, OH: Ohio University Press, 1985). Translation by Noel Barstad with Algis Mickunas.

3. See W. Harman, *op. cit.* D. Elgin, "Awakening Earth: Steps to a Mature Species-Civilization," unpublished manuscript, 1991. P. Russell, *The Global Brain: Speculations on the Evolutionary Leap to Planetary Consciousness* (Los Angeles: J.P. Tarcher, 1983). C. Reich, *The Greening of America* (New York: Random House, 1970). M. Ferguson, *The Aquarian Conspiracy: Personal and Social Transformation in the 1980s* (Los Angeles: J.P. Tarcher, 1980).

PART ONE

THE SEARCH FOR ONENESS AND TRANSCENDENCE

OH, WONDERFUL! OH, WONDERFUL! OH, WONDERFUL!

I AM FOOD. I AM FOOD. I AM FOOD.

I AM THE FOOD-EATER. I AM THE FOOD-EATER.

I AM THE FOOD-EATER.

I AM THE UNITY-MAKER. I AM THE UNITY-MAKER.

I AM THE UNITY-MAKER.

I AM THE FIRST-BORN OF THE WORLD-ORDER (**RITA**),

PRIOR TO THE GODS, IN THE NAVEL OF IMMORTALITY.

HE WHO GIVES ME AWAY, HE INDEED PRESERVES ME.

I, WHO AM FOOD, EAT THE EATER OF FOOD.

I HAVE OVERCOME THE WHOLE WORLD!

TAITTIRIYA-UPANISHAD III.10.6

CHAPTER 1

SPIRITUALITY AND THE MYTHIC STRUCTURE OF CONSCIOUSNESS

CONSCIOUSNESS: THE COMMON DENOMINATOR

The central theme of all spiritual traditions and schools of India is *consciousness*. This is one of the most important points of contact with contemporary Western thought. Since the epoch-making work of Sigmund Freud and C.G. Jung at the threshold of the twentieth century, there has been a steadily growing interest in this fundamental phenomenon of human existence.

At first this rather sudden interest in the nature of consciousness was confined to a narrow circle of psychologists, but before long the general public also began to participate in the rediscovery of this most specifically human dimension. Concepts like "the unconscious," "sublimation," and "archetypes" have long been absorbed into the general vocabulary. In recent years, such notions as "consciousness expansion" and "superconsciousness" were added, not least through the pioneering efforts of transpersonal psychologists. I wish to refer specifically to the work of Ken Wilber, Roger Walsh, Frances Vaughan, and Stanislav Grof—all listed in the bibliography.

Yet only very few people are aware of the far-reaching implications of these and similar psychological concepts. For a positive and fruitful study of Eastern methods of meditative absorption, however, it is indispensable that one should first clarify the functions, limitations, and possibilities of consciousness. This can be done from various angles. The perspective of the present book is that of psychohistory.

PSYCHOHISTORY

Until recently the study of history was an almost exclusively "quantitative" undertaking, dedicated to the accumulation of historical certitudes and only minimally concerned with the psychological dynamics of the respective cultures and societies. It was mainly Arnold Toynbee's monumental work *A Study of History* that paved new ways and prepared the ground for the new discipline of Psychohistory.

Psychohistory was first formally instituted as a comparative historical discipline in its own right at the 1972 Conference of the American Association for the Advancement of Science. The crux of the psychohistoric approach lies in its insight that the contexts and constellations of sociocultural phenomena express definite and definable types of consciousness, and that all transformations in the consciousness substratum are bodied forth in stylistic changes in the diverse domains of cultural life—such as social relationships, art, and philosophy. Thus, history is understood as a consciousness process. This understanding of psychohistory must be distinguished from the psychohistorical studies pursued by psychiatrists whose explorations focus on the individual rather than on history or on the grand structures of a given culture.

It is, above all, the work of the Swiss cultural philosopher Jean Gebser that has helped to inaugurate the new discipline of psychohistory—although Gebser himself did not use this term. The professorial chair especially created for him at the University of Salzburg, Austria, bore the title "Comparative Civilizations."

Through lifelong research, Jean Gebser succeeded in furnishing proof that the history of human civilization is essentially the history of the unfolding of consciousness, and that, as outlined in the Introduction, the evolution of consciousness proceeds in four great mutational leaps: the archaic, the magical, the mythic, and the mental constellations of consciousness.

Gebser's outstanding achievement lies in having pinpointed the characteristics of each structure of consciousness, thereby opening up new vistas of historical understanding. Besides their significance for Psychology, Anthropology, Mythology, Symbology, and Philosophy, his findings are of special importance to all those disciplines that deal with non-Western cultures.

These disciplines largely still operate with the nineteenth-century notion of a monolithic "prelogical mentality." Gebser's much more precise and differentiated model supersedes this outdated notion.

MYTHIC INDIA

For the student of Indian civilization, the mythic structure of consciousness is of particularly great relevance. This is the "frequency" most determinative of Eastern humanity as a whole. Hence we need to state briefly its specific properties.

As Gebser explained, the mythic structure led humanity to an awareness of its internal environment. Just as emotion is the vital medium of the magical consciousness, so imagination (*imago* = picture) or inner experiencing is distinctive of the mythic consciousness. The mythic consciousness is "introvertive" or, as W.S. Haas put it, "centripetal."[1]

With the emergence of the mythic consciousness, the mere associative-analogical thinking peculiar to the magical consciousness was enriched by the appearance of full-fledged symbolic thought, fed by saturated inner vision. This is captured in the word *myth* itself. As Gebser noted:

> Myth is the closing of mouth and eyes; since it is a silent inward gaze (and inner listening), it is essentially a gazing at the psyche, which can be seen and represented as well as heard and made audible. Myth is this representing and making audible; it is the articulation, the report . . . about that which has been seen and heard inwardly.[2]

However, although the ancient Eastern cultures express preeminently the mythic consciousness, they do not lack the capabilities of the mental consciousness. To assume otherwise would be a blatant denial of the very existence of the great philosophies that form an intrinsic part of the Eastern heritage. These philosophies are in no way inferior to those that emerged in Greece about the same time. The metaphysical ideas found in the philosophical portions of the *Rig-Veda* and in the *Upanishads* are as much expressions of the early mental structure of consciousness as are the ideas of Pythagoras, Heraclitus, or Plato—whose philosophies were also strongly tinged by the mythic consciousness.

It was Aristotle, Plato's disciple, who first embodied a style of consciousness somewhat more removed from the mythic matrix. His philosophy in turn dominated Christian scholastic thought until the sixteenth century. In this way, Aristotle can be said to have set the stage for the fateful development of the mental consciousness into its deficient mode—the rational consciousness.

In the East, the mental component did not become so completely divorced from its mythic substratum as has been the case in the West. However, the "Westernization" of the Eastern hemisphere is rapidly changing all this. Western-educated Hindus are apt to be just as locked into the mental-rational consciousness as their European counterparts.

Now the ancient quest for oneness and transcendence can appear to them, too, as quaint and meaningless. Myth can be dismissed as a silly story, or mere phantasy. Traditional mores can be rejected in favor of "enlightened" modern values and attitudes. The result is predictable: psychological isolation, moral confusion, and spiritual denudation.

When we do not properly understand but merely reject the mythic consciousness, we deprive ourselves of the possibility of psychic and social integration. The mythic consciousness is as necessary as the mental consciousness. The same is true of the archaic and the magical consciousness. We can ignore these structures only at our peril.

The mythic consciousness operates on the basis of polarity, or ambivalence. This is evident from its cyclic concept of time and its fascination with the circle. Its style of thought tends to be noncausal, or polar, and its preeminent mental function is the imagination. In its degree of awareness it corresponds to the dream state. Its focus is the psyche, or soul. It articulates itself in envisioned myths and mythology (as spoken myths). Its accentuated bodily organs are the heart and the mouth. It is past-oriented, as epitomized in the widespread practice of ancestor worship. Finally, the mythic consciousness is associated with a pre-perspectival spatial awareness: It does not feel at home in space and time, but clings to the timeless and spaceless eternity.

THE QUEST FOR TRANSCENDENCE

The mythic consciousness, as we encounter it in the spiritual traditions of India, is forever seeking to transcend its inherent spatio-temporal limitations. Its perennial quest for transcendence is the search for a state of flawless existence, marked by absolute stability and unutterable bliss. It endeavors to accomplish this by diving deep into the psychic ocean, pushing through its many layers, and emerging hale on the "other shore."

This process of transcendence involves withdrawal from the ego-bound self in favor of the universal Self, which is experienced as the very ground of existence. Thus authenticity is sought outside the sphere of space and time, in the permanent dimension of absolute reality, or divinity. All psychotechnical methods of Yoga and other similar spiritual traditions, rooted in the mythic consciousness, are designed to escape the mechanisms of the brain and mind, which are bound by time.

The myths surrounding these methods are likewise tools of transcendence. They are intended to create a resonance in the listener by which he or she can slip into the state of timelessness. They not only tell of that state of blissful permanence but actively seek to evoke it. As Joseph Campbell noted, "myths do not come from a *concept* system; they come from a *life* system; they come out of a deep center . . . from where the heart is."[3] And they lead back to it, back to the origin.

Traditionally, myths were not merely told but performed, or reenacted in sacred rituals. Yoga and the other spiritual traditions, by and large, can be looked upon as such rituals by which the aspirant endeavors to return to the transtemporal origin.

MYTHIC AND INTEGRAL CONSCIOUSNESS

Now and then in the history of Indian civilization, however, the vertical thrust toward oneness and transcendence encountered objection. The mythic quest for unity was seen as being needlessly limited, since it excludes the world. This alternative current grew out of spiritual experience rather than abstract theory. Occasionally, some rare individual reached the end of the great mythic journey to the Self only to gain the insight that spiritual development does not end there. The mystical ascent is merely one arc of a circle that comprises also the postmystical return of consciousness to the world.

In other words, after the climactic event of mystical immersion into the transcendental Reality, those sages sought to properly

incarnate their newly won freedom and joy. They returned to the
world, endeavoring to transform, enrich, and ennoble it. Their orientation was integrative, or holistic. Hence they did not deny the
body, the mind, or social relations.

Today an analogous orientation is current in the quest for
wholeness. As philosopher Carl G. Vaught explained, this quest
"moves forward toward a larger, more inclusive unity, but it also
leads us back to the origins of our individual existence."[4] That is to
say, it integrates past and future in the present, and thus is both
mystical and world-affirming. The parallel to the integrative efforts of ancient India is obvious.

The colorful religious and philosophical history of India can
in part be understood as having unfolded through the tension
between the archaic-magical-mythic consciousness seeking transcendence and the holistic aspiration unique to the integral consciousness.

When we consider that the earliest integral breakthroughs occurred more than 2,500 years ago, we cannot but admire the spiritual genius of India. At that time Europe, with the exception of
Greece, was still steeped in the late mythic consciousness. But the
Indian people were not only pursuing their spiritual disciplines
and lofty metaphysics; they were also developing the skills of the
mental structure of consciousness, notably logic.

On the whole, however, logic and philosophy remained sub-
servient to metaphysics. Until modern times, India never lost sight
of the great spiritual ideals formulated by the sages and seers
of the ancient Vedic era. It remained a country of yogins, ascetics,
visionaries, and priests. Hence the empirical sciences did not
develop there beyond the rudimentary stage.

The strength of Indian humanity lies in its exceptional gift for
introspection and mystical realization. It is in the domain of the
psyche and the spirit that the people of India have demonstrated
their greatest ingenuity. It is here that they engaged in their most
daring experiments and, today, have the most significant contribution to make to the emerging global civilization.

Geryke Young's regret that "Asian civilization has contributed
nothing to our modern world, not even a single idea" is unfounded.[5] After all, there is the case of Christianity itself, which

started as a small Eastern cult. It is true, however, that in all essential matters the West as a whole has barely looked to the East for inspiration. In recent decades, discontented Westerners have opened up to Oriental ideas and teachings, and their numbers are steadily increasing; nevertheless, mainstream Western society is still engaged in an unproductive monologue, which now must be broadened into a true dialogue.

East and West, as well as North and South, need each other. Our species can no longer afford to be self-divided. Our future depends on whether we as individuals and as societies can learn—quickly—from the experiences of the different branches of our single human family, and discover how to live in harmony with one another.

NOTES

1. See W.S. Haas, *The Destiny of the Mind: East and West* (London: Faber & Faber, 1956). See also G. Young, *Two Worlds—Not One: Race and Civilization* (London: Ad Hoc Publications, 1969).

2. J. Gebser, *Ursprung und Gegenwart*, p. 77. The English translation is the present author's.

3. J.M. Maher & D. Briggs, *An Open Life: Joseph Campbell in Conversation with Michael Toms* (Burdett, NY: Larson Publications, 1988), p. 21.

4. C.G. Vaught, *The Quest for Wholeness* (Albany, NY: SUNY Press, 1982), p. 4.

5. G. Young, *Two Worlds—Not One*, p. 44.

CHAPTER 2

THE TRANSCENDENCE OF CONSCIOUSNESS

TRANSFORMATION AND TRANSCENDENCE

The spiritual traditions and schools of India, and of anywhere else for that matter, all revolve around the ideal of transcending the ordinary human condition. They offer a great variety of practical means of effecting a deep-level change in consciousness. We cannot radically change our physical shape, but we can extensively restructure our inner world.

Consciousness can be described as the medium by which we experience reality. It is a rather plastic medium, which exists in various states, notably wakefulness, dreaming, deep sleep, and trance. In our society, we tend to overrate the waking state and not take other modes of consciousness seriously enough. However, in traditional societies, the dream state is often considered to be just as important as the waking one. It is thought to give us access to the subtle dimensions of existence.

In the spiritual traditions, many other modes of consciousness are distinguished and described. Broadly speaking, these fall under the category of states of meditation and ecstasy. They are cultivated for the simple reason that they disclose additional aspects or levels of reality, some of which appear to be more fundamental than our everyday physical reality.

Thus, the ascetics or yogins seek to bring about a metamorphosis of their consciousness in order to experience and interact with "higher" (or "deeper") levels of reality. Yoga is the technology of consciousness transformation *par excellence*. Its ideas and techniques, which go back to pre-Buddhist times, have influenced all other traditions of India. Above all, it has been in lively dialogue with Vedanta (the nondualist tradition), which is the predominant metaphysical orientation in ancient and modern India. Sometimes it is difficult to hold these two apart, especially since *yoga* is also a generic term for spiritual discipline *per se*.

I will primarily draw on these two traditions in the following chapters, though I will also make use of Buddhist and Jaina sources. Each school within these diverse traditions has its own understanding of the spiritual process and its own program of personal transformation. They all seek to modify the way we perceive the world. But they also endeavor to accomplish more than that. All in their own way aim not only at the transmutation of consciousness but also at its ultimate *transcendence*. Transformation is seen as a means to transcendence. It is not sought for its own sake.

This emphasis on transcendence represents a significant difference from most schools of modern psychotherapy, which seek to restore a person to "normality" and are chiefly interested in the ordinary waking consciousness and its smooth functioning.

Exceptions to this rule are those transpersonal psychologists who encourage "altered states of consciousness" to promote overall psychic integration. But seldom do they have either the knowledge to supervise, or the means to enhance, the radical path of transcendence pursued in the spiritual traditions.

Transcendence is a slippery term, which has been used in many ways. For instance, human thought can be viewed as a form of transcendence, since it bridges the gulf between the inner and the outer world. Or we can speak of transcendence when we leave behind old habits. But the ascetics and yogins have something more radical in mind. For them, transcendence means the suspension of all ordinary psychic processes and one's awakening as pure, contentless Awareness.

Such transcendence is equivalent to flawless ecstasy. The body-mind is eclipsed by a much larger Awareness. In fact, the spiritual adepts insist that this Awareness is identical with reality. It is not merely a *state* of consciousness. Rather, it is said to exceed all possible modes of perceiving the world. There is only that pure Awareness in which subject and object are perfectly coalesced. It precedes consciousness and its multiple phenomena.

IN PURSUIT OF THE TRANSCENDENTAL SELF

The ultimate unmodifiable Awareness is often referred to as the Self (*purusha, atman*), because it is realized as the irreducible subjective core of the human being. It is that which remains when all the layers upon layers of conscious activity are peeled back. This idea is shared by both Yoga and Vedanta, as well as certain idealistic schools of Buddhism. All those schools of Hinduism that are anchored in the mythic structure of consciousness have the transcendental Self as their ultimate goal. They provide programs for realizing it outside and beyond the phenomenal world. The following words of Vidyaranya, a renowned Vedanta teacher of the fourteenth century, are typical of this approach:

> When the notion of an isolated entity and the notion of an [external] universe are eradicated, then there remains only the innate Self.[1]

The Sanskrit texts of Hinduism are replete with such statements. All the scriptures emphasize the inferior value of mundane existence and exalt the excellence of that luminous Being that abides beyond the realm of the sun and that is imperceptible and unknowable; for, "thither the eye does not extend, nor speech, nor the mind."[2]

This transintelligible universal subject is felt to be the true essence of the human being. At the same time it is held to be the ultimate good, the *summum bonum* of human existence. The existential logic of the ancient Indian sages is here irresistible: If we do recognize that we live in a state of falseness, we must spare no effort to change our situation and regain authenticity by realizing our true identity, which is the Self.

In Classical Yoga, which advocates an extreme dualist metaphysics, the realization of the Self is understood to occur in perfect isolation from the world, including its transcendental core. Self and world are supposed to be forever apart, and only through a process of spiritual ignorance do we experience ourselves as implicated in the world. Upon Self-realization, this delusion is lifted from us, and we—as pure spirit—escape the prison of matter.

Classical Yoga, which was formulated by Patanjali in the second or third century A.D., shares this strange dualism with Classical Samkhya. This latter school was founded by Ishvara Krishna some time in the fourth century A.D. and can be considered a cousin to Patanjali's system.

Vedanta and most other schools of Yoga subscribe to a nondualist metaphysics. The Self is said to be not only our subjective core but also the transcendental foundation of the objective world. Thus, in their ecstasy, the sages frequently exclaimed "*aham brahma asmi*" or "I am the Absolute." The *brahman* is the Ground of existence, the transcendental backdrop against which all the myriad of phenomena arise and vanish again. *Atman* and *brahman* are the same Reality, seen from different angles. The difference between them is merely a mental construct, which has no absolute validity. It is a product of the unenlightened mind, which fragments the perfect continuum that is Reality.

All mythically oriented schools of Hindu spirituality regard the world of phenomena, of multiplicity, as somehow less than real and hence finally undesirable. They strive to simplify and unify existence to the point where it is reduced to that single Self.

THE MYTHIC TREND IN BUDDHISM, VEDANTA, AND YOGA

Even the heretic Gautama, the founder of Buddhism, did not escape this powerful unifying tendency of the mythic structure of consciousness. Where he conspicuously differs from the main stream of India's liberation teachings is in his consistent refusal to speculate about this ultimate Reality. He was so adamant in this attitude that some of his followers and critics believed that he denied the reality of Being as such. If this were true, it would mean that the Buddha taught outright nihilism, which would make nonsense of his "noble eightfold path."

The state of "extinction" (*nirvana*) that he realized and taught is more than the mere transcendence of the phenomenal world with its abundance of suffering. This is evident from a few passages in the Buddhist Pali canon where the Buddha talks in positive terms about the ultimate realization. But on the whole he kept silent, remaining satisfied with pointing the way to that imponderable mystery.

An important aspect of the Buddha's teaching is his doctrine that phenomena lack a stable essence. He spoke of them as being "devoid of self" or "inessential" (*anatman*). It is often held that the Buddha used the term *anatman* in direct opposition to the Vedanta notion of *atman*, or Self. More likely, he introduced it to countermand the popular notion that the body is inhabited by an ego, or permanent entity.[3]

In any case, none of the Buddha's extant sermons states that a transcendental Being does not exist. Rather, this great master's emphasis was on the pragmatics of the spiritual path, which he understood as a way out of the maze of the world. His indifference to metaphysical guesswork not only left ample scope for practical experimentation, but also reduced the danger lurking in nondualist schools of thought—namely, that of false idealism and self-delusion.

Like the Buddha, the founder of Classical Yoga also bears out the powerful influence of the mythic consciousness of unification, which came to dominate the cultural life in India. In contrast to the nondualism of the metaphysical movement of Vedanta, Patanjali appears to have rejected the idea that the ultimate Reality is singular. Instead he postulated a separate subjective core for each entity, which he called *purusha* (literally "man"). This pluralistic conception[4] was the main reason why Classical Yoga and also Classical Samkhya lost in the philosophical competition with the nondualist schools of Vedanta. Metaphysical pluralism is simply not as persuasive a viewpoint.

The mythic spirituality, which is typical of early Buddhism and most schools within the Yoga and Vedanta traditions, is completely oriented toward attaining the premundane-pretemporal Reality. It is based on rigorous introversion and a firm rejection of the world. Not infrequently, this strictly ascetic approach assumes the character of an open flight from the world; then the cosmos is regarded as entirely hostile and evil.

In Advaita Vedanta, the prominent tradition of nondualism, the world-denying orientation is most strikingly expressed in the principal philosophical tenet that the manifold world is merely an illusion (*maya*), or profound distortion of the truth—which is that Reality is singular.

For instance, Shankara, the greatest Vedanta authority of all time, described phenomenal life as a "prison"[5] and the sense objects as "more poisonous than a cobra's venom,"[6] or as "sharks."[7] Admittedly, these quotations are not from one of Shankara's philosophical works but from a popular didactic poem attributed to him. Nevertheless, they are indicative of Shankara's great yearning for Being (*sat*) and his fundamental distrust of all Becoming (*bhava*).

We may see in Shankara the incarnate idea of the mythic consciousness, which is ever ready to renounce the Many in favor of the One. The Self was his lifelong concern as a thinker and preacher. According to Hindu tradition, he had realized it at the young age of twelve. He was thus not merely a learned man but a spiritual adept.

It appears that in his youth Shankara was a follower of Classical Yoga. This is suggested by an extant Sanskrit commentary on the *Yoga-Sutra*, entitled *Vivarana*, which was apparently authored by him.[8] Subsequently he converted to Vedanta. True to his yogic background, he lived as a monk all his life. Although he wrote numerous scholastic and popular works and traveled widely in India, his basic outlook was that of renunciation. The world held no hope for him.

THE REDUCTION OF CONSCIOUSNESS

As already indicated, the primary agent of the spiritual process is consciousness. From the mythic perspective, it is viewed as the shadowlike imitation of the transcendental Awareness and as the underlying cause of our perception of an external world. In the Vedanta system, consciousness is plainly defined as a "reflection of the transcendental Awareness" (*cid-abhasa*). Thus, a distinction is made between *citta* (consciousness) and *cit* (pure Awareness).

In the ordinary waking state, we identify with consciousness and hence are typically at the mercy of its functions (i.e., sensations, emotions, thoughts, etc.). The goal of mythic spirituality is to dismantle this false identity by restricting these activities of consciousness. First, we must reduce our sensory intake, thus creating a distance from the objective world. Then we must progressively empty our internal universe.

This process leads to a threshold where a sudden abrupt break takes place that throws us into pure Being-Awareness, our true identity. This realization is explained as the achievement of autonomy or emancipation, which is variously called *moksha*, *mukti, apavarga*, or *kaivalya*. As we will see, it is also referred to as "immortality."

The yogic process of deconstruction is aptly described in the *Kshurika-Upanishad* ("Secret Doctrine of the Knife"), where the yogin is instructed to "slice" his consciousness from his body, member by member. As soon as the empirical consciousness is without any support, it collapses—and thus creates "space" for the transcendental Awareness to become evident. To put it differently, the emptied consciousness turns out to be infinite Being-Awareness.

Perhaps these metaphysical intricacies can best be grasped when one understands the ordinary consciousness as a *process of becoming* conscious, rather than as a thing, as we tend to do. This incessant "becoming" of consciousness is nowhere analyzed more acutely than in Buddhism. Unlike the Hindu sages, who couched their mystical experiences in idealistic terms, the Buddhist monastics were realists with a keen interest in psychological analysis. They penetrated deep into the nature of phenomenal existence in order to gain greater insight into the laws governing our inner life.

The intellectual efforts of these sharp-witted Buddhist pragmatists are found condensed in the doctrine of the "bearers" (*dharma*), which are the ultimate building blocks of space-time and consciousness. Buddhologist Edward Conze once remarked about this theory that it would cause considerable emotional difficulties to anyone who had not yet developed the virtue of dispassion, "because it deprives objects of all basis for sensory gratification, fear, love, hope and tribal sentiments."[9]

The *dharmas* occur in combinations that light up for an infinitesimal fraction of a second only to give way to new dharma aggregations, which have the same short destiny. According to a well-known classification, these combinations are arranged into five groups, called *skandha*, as follows:

1. the material (*rupa*);
2. sensation (*vedana*);

3. perception (*samjna*);
4. mental impulses (*samskara*), and
5. consciousness (*vijnana*).

There is no direct causal relationship between the dharmas, but their arising is governed by a conditional nexus that is regulated by the totality of conditions responsible for the occurrence of new dharma conglomerations. This is a striking example of systems thinking in antiquity.

The purpose of this analytical model is to shatter and eradicate such notions as "self," "ego," "person," "doer," and so on, all of which represent fatal misconceptions. The reduction of the inner and outer cosmos to impermanent suprapersonal events is meant to drive home the utter transiency of the phenomenal reality and to spur on those who have entered the path to enlightenment. The dharma doctrine is as much a model as it is a method, a radical technique of introversion and transcendence.

The dharma teaching is a doctrine of hope. For when the ever-rotating "wheel of becoming" (*bhava-cakra*) comes to a standstill in one's own case, we discover authentic existence. That this existence is not merely a state of unconsciousness is evident from the designation *buddha*, by which the founder of Buddhism referred to himself and others like him. It means "he who has awakened." The adept who has recovered his true identity has not sunk to the level of inert matter but is enlightened. Enlightenment is the same as the supreme Being-Awareness.

Possibly the most concise formulation of this process of emptying followed by the manifestation of the transcendental Self is given by Patanjali in his *Yoga-Sutra* (I.2–3):

> Yoga is the restriction of the activity of consciousness.—
> [When consciousness is appeased], then the "seer" [i.e., the Self] abides [in its] own form.

Extracted from its various doctrinal and terminological coverings, the central idea expressed here is relatively simple: We are other than what we generally believe ourselves to be. Our habitual identification with a particular body and mind is due to an inexplicable metaphysical blindness. This spiritual myopia is at the root of all our ills. If we desire to "come to ourselves," that is, to become what we in essence already are, we must remove this innate error or misconception and cease to identify with what higher knowledge reveals to be foreign to our true identity, the splendorous Being-Awareness.

NOTES

1. *Panca-Dashi* VI.12b.

2. *Kena-Upanishad* I.3.

3. See E. Conze, *Buddhist Thought in India* (London: Allen & Unwin, 1962), p. 36.

4. In the *Yoga-Sutra* there is no clearcut statement of Patanjali's position on the singularity or plurality of the transcendental subject. However, his Sanskrit commentators are agreed that he taught the latter.

5. *Viveka-Cudamani,* verse 272.

6. *Ibid.,* verse 77.

7. *Ibid.,* verse 80.

8. This is denied by some Hindu scholars, but the German Indologist Paul Hacker has made a good case in support of this attribution.

9. E. Conze, *Buddhist Thought in India,* p. 103.

CHAPTER 3

UNIFICATION AS A BIPOLAR PROCESS

IMMORTALITY AND FREEDOM

Spiritual transcendence can be characterized in different ways—as Self-realization, God-realization, perfection, wholeness, liberation, freedom, unbounded bliss, and immortality. We encounter all these terms in the Sanskrit literature. Perhaps the two most commonly used terms are "liberation" and "immortality." Whereas the former designation is from the viewpoint of the mythic structure of consciousness, the latter expresses a longing pertaining to the magical structure.

Immortality, the older of the two terms, originally signified deathlessness in the heavens—a religious conviction that corresponds well with the world-oriented magical consciousness. For the pious men and women of the Vedic age, the death of the physical frame coincided with the soul's triumphant entry into the blessed abode of the gods. That abode was thought to have spatial extension, with its own geography. Entrance into heaven meant eternal life in undiminishable bliss.

Only those who during their life on earth had ignored the gods and neglected to perform the daily sacrifice, the food of the immortals, could be expected to be hurled into the dark abyss of hell. In the Vedic era, which extended from roughly 2000 to 1000 B.C., the later-prominent idea of repeated incarnations on earth had as yet not been formulated. A person's post-mortem fate appears to have been either untold happiness in the company of the gods or eternal agony in hell.

The Sanskrit word for "immortality" is *amrita*, which is a composite of the negative prefix *a-* and the perfect passive participle of the verb "to die" (*mri*). It thus means literally "not died," that is, "immortal." In the course of time the expression amrita came to signify the "nectar of immortality" known to mythology.

The classic instance of this specific shade of meaning can be found in what is perhaps the most popular story of the *Mahabharata* epic: the myth of the churning of the ocean. This tale is a perfect example of the yogic or introspective origin of many of India's myths. It sheds wonderful light on the perennial spiritual endeavor to gain access to the invisible domain of the gods. The following is a brief summary of this myth.

The gods once conferred with each other about how they could come into possession of the celestial nectar of immortality, which had vanished during the previous period of cosmic dissolution. Narayana, the Creator, advised them to churn the world ocean with the help of the demons in order to retrieve the divine ambrosia.

The gods enlisted Ananta, the king of the serpent race, to uproot the sacred world mountain so that it could be used as a twirling-stick. The back of the ruler of the tortoises served as a fulcrum point for the mountain. Ananta wound his serpent body around the dislodged *axis mundi*, and the gods gripped the tail-end of it, while the demons got hold of Ananta's head. Then the two parties pulled the giant body rhythmically to and fro, thus rotating the mountain.

Soon the water of the cosmic ocean began to sizzle and steam, giving birth to all kinds of entities and objects. However, the waters did not yield the hoped-for nectar. Gods and demons resigned from exhaustion. Again they approached Narayana, begging him for his support, which was promptly given. With new strength they proceeded with their task. The ocean bubbled up under their furious churning. Many strange creatures emerged from the raging sea, and finally the celestial physician Dhanyantari appeared, holding a white bowl in his hands which contained the nectar.

All of a sudden the world ocean vomited huge masses of poisonous liquid that threatened to spread over the entire world. To save the universe from total destruction, God Shiva, the lord of yogins and ascetics, gulped down the poison, which turned his throat blue but otherwise failed to harm him. The demons did not let this unique opportunity slip by, but quickly stole the nectar.

However, quarreling over their booty, they failed to sip from the celestial draught and thus gain once and for all supreme

dominion over the created universe. Again through the interven-
tion of Narayana, who assumed a female shape causing considerable confusion among the demons, the duped gods recaptured the
nectar of immortality. A fierce battle ensued from which the gods
emerged as victors.[1]

THE FLIGHT TO LIBERATION

In contrast to "immortality," the term "liberation" carries the
stamp of the mythic consciousness, which regards the path to enlightenment as leading away from everything that is worldly and
impermanent. The Sanskrit word *moksha*, meaning "emancipation" or "release," is already to be found quite frequently in the
ancient hymns of the *Rig-Veda*. However, in that early scripture, it
is employed almost exclusively in the sense of "setting free from
sin (*papa*) or transgression."[2] As such it refers to a psychological
process rather than a transcendental realization. The term acquired
its classic meaning of "liberation" with the emergence of the secret
doctrines given out in the *Upanishads*, literary compositions dating
back to the ninth century B.C.

Traditionally, there are said to be 108 *Upanishads*, though their
actual number exceed two hundred, and works bearing this hon-
orable title are still being written. What they have in common is a
nondualist metaphysics, which entails a practical path of transcendence. The goal is liberation either at the end of this lifetime or
while still inhabiting a physical body.

What fascinates and entices ascetics of the mythic structure of
consciousness is not so much the thought that the eradication of all
sin will transport them to the delightful mansions of the gods, but
the insight that the abolishment of their spiritual nescience eman-
cipates them from the fetters of conditioned existence as such.
They are happy to renounce the promises of heaven for the realization of the Unconditioned.

In subsequent times, the terms "immortality" and "liberation," originally standing for completely different experiences and
attitudes, came to be equated. Both were freely used to symbolize
the deathless freedom of the ultimate Being.

The path to liberation, or enlightenment, is a path of progressive simplification. The adepts seek to withdraw from multiplicity,

rather like a bird takes off from a many-branched tree into the sun-lit single sky. Since time immemorial, adepts have been likened to birds. Thus shamans are thought to be able to leave the material realm for higher worlds by transferring their consciousness to a subtle body. But in the case of great spiritual masters, the bird metaphor is applicable for another reason. For they rise above the world—morally and spiritually.

PRACTICE AND DISPASSION

The two wings that carry the adept safely to the "other shore" are the practice of unification and the renunciation of the Many. The respective Sanskrit terms are *abhyasa* ("practice") and *vairagya* ("dispassion"). In Vyasa's *Yoga-Bhashya* ("Speech on Yoga"), the oldest extant commentary on the Yoga aphorisms of Patanjali, the harmonious functioning of these two poles of any spiritual path is expressed in the following way:

> The stream of consciousness flows in both [directions]. It flows to the good, and it flows to the bad. The one commencing with discernment and terminating in liberation (*kaivalya*) flows to the good. The one commencing with lack of discernment and terminating in conditioned existence flows to the bad. Through dispassion one's flowing out to the [transient] sense objects is checked, and through the practice of the vision of discernment, the stream of discernment is laid bare. Thus the restriction of the activity of consciousness is dependent upon both.[3]

The *Bhagavad-Gita* ("Lord's Song") likewise draws attention to the importance and complementary nature of practice and dispassion. In one stanza (VI.35), Lord Krishna says to his disciple Prince Arjuna:

> The mind, O strong-armed one, is undoubtedly unsteady and difficult to control. Yet through practice and dispassion . . . it can be seized.

That both means must be practiced together in order to effect the "flight" to the transcendental Self is also confirmed by

Shankara, the author of *Viveka-Cudamani* ("Crest-Jewel of Discernment"). He states:

> Dispassion and insight [cultivated through the practice of unification] are like the wings of a bird for the aspirant. . . . Without the help of these two, the creeper [called] "emancipation," which climbs to the summit of the [world-]edifice, cannot be reached.[4]

The symbolism of "flight" is found already in the three-thousand-year-old *Panca-Vimsha-Brahmana* (V.I.10). Here the sacrificer, who for all practical purposes can be identified with the yogin or ascetic who performs the "inner" sacrifice, is described as a bird that rises heavenward. An echo of this idea is found in the *Mahabharata* epic (XII.326.31), where we can read: "Like a bird rising from the abyss [of this world], he attains infinity in the next [world]." This symbolism is equally at home in Hindu, Buddhist, and Jaina scriptures.

The birdlike nature of spiritual practitioners consists in their conquest of gravity, both internally and externally. Their spiritual striving uplifts and frees them from the karmic effects of their material life. Their destiny is no longer governed by the causal processes of the world, where everyone harvests the fruits of their moral and immoral volitions and actions. An adept's karma is neither white nor black, but neutral.

More than that, all the traditions insist that these adepts also rise above the physical laws of Nature. Thus, they are said to possess the psychic power (*siddhi*) of levitation, which is the capacity to literally rise above the world. Because the great adepts have conquered the transcendental "ether"—the boundless space of consciousness—they also acquire unconditional mastery over matter, which is merely a condensed form of that subtle ether.

In other words, their mysterious powers of levitation and telekinesis are simply expressions on the physical level of the adepts' transcendental "flight." The phenomenon of levitation is perhaps the most symbolic of all the magical achievements attributed to adepts (*siddha*). They do not experience the body as dead, dragging matter but as a vast storehouse of consciousness-energy, capable of incredible transformations.

The last sentence hints at the cathartic aspect of the path to emancipation. Spiritual life is not only a comprehensive process of unification, it is also a systematic catharsis. Purity, gnostic knowledge, and magical power are concepts that are, as the Italian Indologist Corrado Pensa has shown, organically related in any system of spiritual practice.[5]

The word *abhyasa*, introduced above, designates the practice pole of the spiritual path. It does not occur in the older strata of the Hindu literature, where, in its place, the term *shrama* or "exertion" is chiefly used. The word *abhyasa* makes its first appearance in the *Bhagavad-Gita*[6] and the *Shvetashvatara-Upanishad*[7]. These two works belong to approximately the fourth century B.C.

The term *abhyasa* is composed of the prefix *abhi* or "unto" and *as-a* or "sitting," thus meaning a "sitting for" or "applying oneself to" something. In secular contexts, it is commonly used in the sense of "repetition." This usage is telling, for practice in principle is just that: disciplined repetition. As aptly put by Yoga master Patanjali:

> Practice is the [repeated] effort to stabilize [consciousness].—However, it [gains] firm ground [only when it] is cultivated for a long time, uninterruptedly, and attentively.[8]

"Practice" stands for the concentrated inner application to the realization of the transcendental Being. It consists in the careful discrimination between the real and the unreal, the permanent and the impermanent. Implicit in this is the idea that the real, or permanent, is ultimately desirable, whereas the transient is, in the last analysis, unworthy of human motivation. Such subtle discrimination is the foundation of spiritual inwardness and unification.

The word *vairagya*, literally "dispassion," also belongs to the vocabulary of the second half of the first millennium B.C. It is a synonym of *viraga*, which is widely used in Buddhism. It denotes the same as *vitrishna* ("thirstlessness"), *tyaga* ("abandoning"), and *samnyasa* ("renunciation"). All these words refer to the ascetic turning away from worldly objects and values. However, it is important to make a clear distinction between purely internal renunciation and actual physical abandonment of mundane life. Mythic Yoga only knows the latter type of dispassion.

THE INTERPLAY OF UNITIVE STRIVING
AND RENUNCIATION

At the outset of the yogic path the emphasis lies understandably on the positive or practice pole. Nevertheless, dispassion is not wholly lacking. Even the resolve to take upon oneself the yoke of a disciplined course of action presupposes a certain measure of inner distance from the turmoil of mundane life. However, the readiness of the novice to renounce worldly pleasures bears no comparison with the consummate thirstlessness of the adepts. This is clear from the fact that the accomplished master is typically said to transcend both good and evil, whereas struggling students are subject to the moral law of causation (*karma*). Hence they are expected to live by rather strict rules.

Practice without dispassion is conducive to ego inflation and hunger for power and thus increased entanglement in things worldly. Dispassion without practice, on the other hand, is like a blunt knife: The psychosomatic energies generated by abdicating from the world remain without an outlet and at best cause confusion in body and mind. Both poles need to be cultivated simultaneously and with prudence. Indolence and lack of circumspection instantly thwart all one's efforts.

The interdependence of practice and dispassion is a recurring theme in the *Yoga-Vasishtha*, which is the most fascinating and versatile work on nondualist Yoga. Vidyaranya, who in his *Jivan-Mukti-Viveka* constantly quotes from this mammoth work, refers to one passage which describes the gradual transformation of the yogin's aspirations. The following is a paraphrase of it:

Half of the aspirations of those who have not as yet made any noticeable progress may be given to the fulfillment of material desires, one fourth to the study of the sacred tradition, and the remaining fourth to their dedication to the teacher. Those who have progressed a little should give only one fourth to the fulfillment of their desires, half to their dedication to the teacher, and the last fourth to the truths of the sacred tradition. Those who have climbed to the heights of Yoga should dedicate themselves equally to contemplation and renunciation.[9]

Vidyaranya, himself obviously an experienced adept, recommends the following time schedule:

1. exercises (meditation, etc.)   1/2 hour
2. sitting at the feet of the teacher   1 hour
3. rest   1 hour
4. study of the sacred texts   1 hour
5. exercises   1 hour

After this cycle, students may take up their daily duties and carry them out in an appropriate frame of mind. This program should be gradually prolonged until it occupies the practitioner's whole life. This endorsement of a step-by-step adoption of spiritual practice is a compromise with more radical forms of mythic spirituality, which demand that ascetics cast off the burdens of social life there and then. Vidyaranya's more balanced approach is explained by his acceptance of the brahmanical doctrine of life stages (*ashrama*). Their principle is as follows.

Ideally a man's life should proceed in four hierarchical stages. From birth to the marriageable age, a man belongs to the student stage (*brahmacarya*). Thereafter he enters the stage of the householder (*garhasthya*). When the first signs of ageing appear and he has conscientiously fulfilled his duties toward his family and society, he should retire to the solitude of the forest. This is the stage of the forest dweller (*vana-prasthya*). During the last quarter of his life, he may adopt the stage of the wandering ascetic (*samnyasa*). Then, having reached the apex of spiritual life, he may live in the continuous actualization of the supreme Being-Awareness.

A similar life pattern applies to women. They were traditionally expected to follow their husbands into retirement and even death. However, India's cultural history is filled with exceptions to this rule. There were, for instance, great women sages who never married or who renounced the world and their marriage before their husbands were ready to follow suit.

At any rate, the model of the stages of life was introduced by Hindu legislators to countermand the ever-present tendency to abandon social obligations and to take refuge in caves and forests. It was an attempt to make the householder existence acceptable to the people at large. Yet, those who were moved to renounce the world seldom waited for the right social moment, and they were no less accepted for their extremism. If anything, people admired them for their austerity and capacity for renunciation.

NOTES

1. See *Mahabharata* I.17.5ff.

2. See S. Rohde, *Deliver us from Evil: Studies on the Vedic Ideas of Salvation* (Lund, 1946).

3. *Yoga-Bhashya* I.12.

4. *Viveka-Cudamani*, verse 374.

5. C. Pensa, "On the purification concept in Indian tradition, with special regard to Yoga," *East and West*, new series, XIX (Rome, 1969).

6. *Bhagavad-Gita* VI.35,44; VIII.8; XII.9,10,12; XVII.36.

7. *Shvetashvatara-Upanishad* I.14.

8. *Yoga-Sutra* I.13–14.

9. *Jivan-Mukti-Viveka*, Chapter III. I have so far not succeeded in locating these stanzas in the *Yoga-Vasishtha*.

CHAPTER 4

LIFE IS SUFFERING

AWAKENING TO SORROW

The ascetical flight from the world is prompted by the perception of life as suffering. When the mythic consciousness crystallized, humanity made a troubling discovery. Not only did our forebears begin to be self-conscious about their inner life, it also dawned on them that to be alive means to be exposed to an endless round of pain and frustration. The experience of pain was of course nothing new; but with the emergence of the mythic consciousness, humanity for the first time began to experience it doubly—as an unpleasant physical sensation and as emotional distress.

The protégés of the early magical structure of consciousness as yet knew nothing of the heavy burden of a conscious relationship between individual and environment. They still slumbered largely in the safety of the archaic unity-consciousness from which they would emerge, now and then, only to face a world of immense complexity and interconnectedness. The world was for them full of inexplicable happenings and hardly inspired confidence or a feeling of security. But their self-awareness was still too dim to allow them to reflect on this fact or to consciously determine their actions in light of deliberate metaphysical thought. Also, their pain threshold was much higher, and they were relatively free from stress, having a healthy flight-or-fight instinct.

Since the earliest days, humanity has known its share of pain and discomfort. Yet, psychic suffering was the dowry of the mythic consciousness. Just as the incumbents of the magical consciousness experienced the world as veiled and compelling, so those of the mythic structure of consciousness perceived it in its terrifying magnitude and fateful interlinking. This understanding grew ever more acute as humans reached new levels of self-awareness.

The nascent feeling of individuality taking our ancestors from the magical to the mythic consciousness led them to experience themselves as a skiff tossed on the waves of the shoreless ocean of psychic and external events. They searched for a secure berth, but saw everywhere only indefatigable movement, a monotonous coming and going of events. This experience of the continuous flux of phenomena, unfolding in cycles, underlies the mythic vision of the sorrowful nature of human existence.

With the mental structure of consciousness, this knowledge of the pervasive nature of suffering found ample articulation in philosophical teachings. These can be seen as attempts to make sense of suffering, to find reasonable causes for it, and thus to further convert the experience of pain and distress into symbolic forms. If religion, as Karl Marx would have it, is opium for the masses, then philosophy is the sedative for the elite. Both seek to lend meaning to life and to the prevalence of suffering, notably the distress caused by the prospect of individual extinction.

In Europe, Plato gave expression to this sensitivity to suffering when he stated in his *Gorgias* that "life is terrible" (*deinòs o bíos*). Jesus' suffering and violent death were immediately interpreted as a vicarious atonement for the shortcomings (sin) of humanity as a whole, and thus an indirect plea for the reduction of suffering in human life. Today, two thousand years later, bumper stickers reiterate in street idiom the same message: "Life sucks and then you die."

The East had its own apostles of suffering. The omnipresence of suffering preached by India's sages is not merely the pain suffered from the scorching midday sun or the agony caused at the hand of the enemy. These are mere manifestations of the great reality of cosmic suffering. What disconcerts them is the flawed nature of finite existence itself, epitomized in the transiency of life, which they compare to an unsteady dew drop on a leaf. Perhaps the following guiding words of the Buddha best illustrate this instinct of the mythic consciousness, which everywhere ferrets out the trail of suffering.

> This, monks, is the noble truth of suffering: Birth is sorrowful, old age is sorrowful, illness is sorrowful, death is sorrowful, grief, distress and despair are sorrowful; to be united with what is unwanted is sorrowful, to be separated from what is wanted is sorrowful, not to obtain what is desired is sorrowful; in short: the five "groups" (*skandha*) are sorrowful.[1]

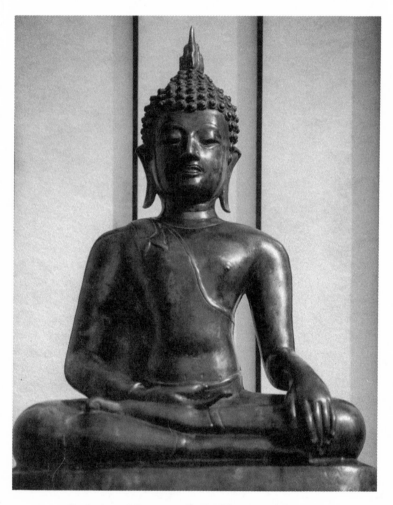

*Sculpture of Gautama the Buddha, one of the great
enlightened masters of the ancient world.*

Even everything that appears as pleasant to the unenlightened mind is steeped in suffering, for does it not harbor anxiety about its loss? Behind every pleasure lurk twenty painful experiences, as Sufi wisdom has it. For the Buddhist, conditioned existence has three characteristics; it is sorrowful (*duhkha*), nonessential (*anatman*), and utterly impermanent (*anitya*).

This view of the universality of suffering is shared by all other spiritual traditions of India. The *Yoga-Sutra* (II.15), for instance, contains this aphorism:

> By reason of the sorrowfulness of the changes [in one's consciousness], the afflictions [of life], and the impressions [in the depth of one's psyche], as well as owing to the disharmony in the activity of the constituents [of Nature itself]—to the discerning [sage] everything is but suffering.

Vyasa, who composed a penetrating commentary on Patanjali's aphorisms, compares the student of Yoga to an eyeball, which is supersensitive. Even a tiny granule of sand causes vehement pain.[2] The more one is able to see things as they really are, the more acute the insight becomes that there is nothing in this world that is not limited, subject to change, and hence ultimately unfulfilling.

Existence means suffering. This is echoed in all esoteric schools and systems. Thus the *Acaranga-Sutra* (I.6.2), a Jaina canonical work, states:

> All beings . . . [experience] their own [short-lived] pleasure and [much] displeasure, pain, great terror, and unhappiness. Everywhere beings are filled with alarm from all directions.

Suffering is the starting-point for the liberation teachings. Hence the manuals frequently commence with a statement of the universal fact of suffering, as for example in the opening verse of Ishvara Krishna's *Samkhya-Karika*, a work belonging to the fourth century A.D. Here we read:

> By reason of the blows of the threefold suffering, [there arises] an inquiry into the means for abolishing this [suffering].

Suffering is said to be threefold because it is (1) either caused

by oneself, or (2) is due to external circumstances, or else (3) derives from supranatural causes. The Sanskrit terms reserved for
these three categories are *adhyatmika* or "subjective," *abhibhautika*
or "environmental," and *adhidaivika* or "destined." This last term
refers to interventions "from above," be it the influence of the stars
or nonhuman discarnate entities who interfere with our lives.

LIFE AS WHEEL AND JUNGLE

The notion of the omnipotence of suffering is intimately associated with another prominent mythical motif, namely that of the
"wheel of life" (*samsara-mandala* or *-cakra*). On one side, it is meant
to depict the interlinkedness of existence and on the other, it portrays the cyclic movement or periodicity of all phenomena, as seen
from the mythic perspective. *Samsara* signifies the world of
change, of the uninterrupted flux of events that roll on, propelled
by karma.

In Tibetan Buddhism, the wheel of existence (*bhava-cakra*) is
depicted with Yama, the Lord of Death, clutching its circumference
in his clawlike fingers and his fangs. It is an image designed to in-
still in the beholder a sense of sobriety, if not fear. The overpower-
ing presence of Yama symbolizes the impermanence of all life—including the long life attributed to the deities of the Buddhist pan-
theon. For life is a wheel that inexorably grinds away all creatures,
good and bad alike. As Paul Brunton observed astutely:

> The West thinks life is a ladder; the East knows it is a
> wheel. The West regards it as a climb, the East as a round-
> about. The West sees a distant perfection towards which we
> progress and develop and evolve. The East sees that escape
> from the wheel can occur now or at any time. The West gives a
> beginning and so must give an end to the ladder. The East sees
> no beginning and no end in a circle.[3]

When we moderns speak of the city as a jungle, we capture
precisely the Eastern sentiment, though the symbol of the jungle
applies not merely to urban life but to finite existence as such. The
Mahabharata epic (XI.5) contains a striking allegory that is worth
relating in this connection.

Once a brahmin went astray in a lush jungle abounding in

dangerous animals and plants, which would have terrified even Yama, the Lord of Death. Little wonder that the poor brahmin was seized with panic. However much he tried to hew himself a path out of the thicket, he only succeeded in getting deeper and deeper into it. Looking up, he realized that the jungle was covered with an impenetrable net, beyond which he glimpsed a giant female with outstretched arms. Five-headed serpent monsters loomed in the sky.

Then the terrified brahmin fell into a pit that had been concealed with brushwood. Hanging upside down with his legs entangled in the shrubbery, he saw a gigantic serpent at the bottom of the pit and a huge elephant with six heads and twelve legs near the opening. Enormous bees swarmed around him, and the honey that trickled from their honeycombs dripped into the brahmin's mouth, increasing his thirst.

Black-and-white rats were gnawing at the tree near the edge of the pit, and it was clear to him that before long he would be crushed under its weight. Almost out of his mind with fear, and without any hope of rescue, he nevertheless still desired to continue his pitiable existence.

This nightmarish picture, which has its parallels in medieval European thought, is a portrayal of the world in its whole absurdity and insidiousness as experienced by the mythic consciousness. The jungle of course represents life, and the ferocious beasts are symbols of the diseases and misfortunes that can befall us. The giant female stands for the transiency of life. The pit is the human body. The serpent in it represents time. The brushwood in which the brahmin got entangled is our greed for existence.

The elephant represents the year, his six heads and twelve legs depicting the six Indian seasons and twelve months respectively. The rats that gnaw at the tree of life are the days and nights, messengers of death. The bees are our desires, and the honey drops symbolize the transient joys that derive from their fulfillment.

FROM SUFFERING TO WISDOM

Because of portrayals like the above allegory, Indian thought has repeatedly been stamped as thoroughly pessimistic. This verdict is precipitate and quite unjustified. It possibly springs from an intellectualist bias against non-Western traditions. Can there be any greater optimism than the conviction of India's sages that we are inherently free and capable of extricating ourselves from the mire of this world through our own effort and will? This unshakeable belief in human freedom is the pivot of all the great teachings of Hinduism, Buddhism, and Jainism. Nihilistic despair, which appears to be a regular feature of the Western rational consciousness, was a rare occurrence on India's soil.

Suffering should rightly be an incentive to remove one's conditionality and enmeshment in sorrowful and transient things. Countless passages in scriptures belonging to very different traditions and eras bear witness to this radical optimism. For instance, the *Markandeya-Purana* (XXXIX.2) plainly states that "knowledge springs from sorrow"—an assurance that is repeated in the *Mahabharata* (III.2.24).

It is in this light that we must understand the observation in the ancient *Brihad-Aranyaka-Upanishad* (V.II) that "illness is the highest asceticism that one can endure." We would be mistaken if we were to see in this statement a parallel to certain interpretations of Christian ethics. The most renowned sages and ascetics of India, like Jesus, never advised to actively seek out suffering. Instead, they taught that suffering is an integral aspect of human life, which we must meet creatively rather than with either a defeatist or a masochistic attitude.

Moreover, all the great schools of Indian esotericism are agreed that suffering does not originate in a supreme cosmic agent. It is an experience that occurs at the intersection between subject and object: in the individual human psyche, which interprets the input which the senses receive from the world.

The true birthplace of suffering is our spiritual blindness (*avidya*) or, as the Jainas call it, "falsity" (*mithyatva*). When this nescience is removed, pain and suffering lose their sting. "He who knows the Self, traverses sorrow," confirms the ancient *Chandogya-Upanishad* (VII.I.3). In other words, Self-realization is the only antidote to our involvement in suffering, life's toxic waste.

The world cannot rid itself of its fundamental nature. It will always be finite and changeable. The wheel will continue to turn forever, or at least until the entire cosmic machinery comes to a standstill. According to Hindu metaphysics, the cosmos will definitely collapse but, after countless eons, it will again spring forth from the Uncreate. This idea has been revived by modern cosmologists.

Our individual lives are most minute events in this cosmic drama. When we contemplate our own finitude against the vast backdrop of the world's billions of years of existence, we are filled with awe, uncertainty, and anxiety. Unless we are aware of our larger spiritual destiny, we are apt to succumb to our fears. Then we typically become desolate and seek to fill our days with substitute realities—all the many gods to which our materialistic civilization pays tribute.

A wiser route, and the only route to fulfilling our true destiny, is that of transcending the fear of death and the fear of life by transcending our encapsulated sense of identity. That is to say, we must exercise our intrinsic freedom to go beyond the human condition and *become* the inconceivable Identity underlying the cosmos at large. This is precisely the grand ideal held before us by the spiritual traditions of India. In the mythic traditions, this ideal is associated with ascetic denial of the world and a somewhat one-sided rejection of the pain and suffering of ordinary life.

The ascetic prefers to engage in suffering of a different type, which is the whole ordeal of a self-denying lifestyle. Asceticism is the deliberate frustration of one's natural tendencies. From the viewpoint of the ascetic, of course, what we deem natural is quite artificial. For the ascetic, ordinary life is unnatural because it ignores our true identity, which is the Self, and instead glorifies the ego. The ego, however, *is* suffering. Hence the path to bliss beyond all sorrow is by way of the transcendence of the ego and its world.

NOTES

1. *Mahavagga* I.6.19.

2. See *Yoga-Bhashya* II.15.

3. P. Brunton, *The Orient: Its Legacy to the West* (Burdett, NY: Larson Publications, 1987), pp. 35-36. This is volume 10 of *The Notebooks of Paul Brunton*.

CHAPTER 5

ESCAPING THE CYCLE OF LIFE AND DEATH

MULTIPLE BIRTHS AND DEATHS

The belief that our life on earth is the only one we have is almost exclusive to our materialistic Western civilization. Most traditional cultures entertain the view that we are visitors here on earth, and that our present visit is neither our first nor our last.[1] Rather, they believe that existence is a continuous switching from one level of being to another—from physical embodiment to a nonphysical state and back to the material plane. In the tenth-century *Yoga-Vasishtha* (V.71.65 and 67), this is expressed as follows:

> A dead [person] is said to have gone [for good], but this is untrue and false. Having become separated from space and time, one experiences [a different level of reality].

> Having cast off [the physical body], the person steeped in desires (*vasana*) assumes a [new] body, just as a monkey in the forest swings from one tree to another.

Thus, what we fear as death is also a birth. We die to one level of existence only to awaken on another. This is in due course followed by our death on the subtle plane, which coincides with our rebirth onto the material level of existence. Birth and death are like a revolving door.

For the mythic consciousness, this prospect of repeated births and deaths is absolutely terrifying. It is the most concrete expression of suffering. For we are constantly being recycled through this uninterrupted series of incarnations, which subjects us to repeated painful experiences in life after life.

The doctrine of reincarnation can be regarded as one of the two great pillars that support the cultural life of traditional India. The second pillar is the conviction that we have the innate capacity to transcend that fateful process. This is the ideal of liberation.

The belief in reembodiment is hinted at for the first time in the older *Upanishads*. It formed part of their secret teaching. However, a few hymns of the ancient *Rig-Veda* seem to indicate that the Sanskrit-speaking tribes of Northern India in fact knew about reincarnation much earlier. If they did not bring this belief with them from their alleged homeland in Russia, they certainly encountered it in India.[2] According to the consensus of scholarly opinion, the Vedic peoples had some notion of it, but the full-fledged teaching of reembodiment had been elaborated by the original inhabitants of the Indian peninsula.

Be that as it may, the sages whose wisdom is crystallized in the *Upanishads* were important catalysts for the dissemination of this eschatological belief within the budding Hindu society. After the eighth century B.C., the doctrine of reincarnation began to exercise a growing influence on the orthodox circles within Hinduism. Henceforth it is found firmly wedded to the doctrine of liberation. This is also true of the traditions of Buddhism and Jainism.

The basic idea behind this archaic teaching is as follows. Our deeds or, according to a more sophisticated version, our volitions determine the quality of our future existence. Wholesome acts or volitions lead to favorable future states (rebirths), whereas unwholesome acts or volitions result in unfavorable states. Thus, reward and punishment are meted out according to an implacable law of moral causation, which is an integral aspect of Nature—the law of karma.

The Sanskrit word *karma* literally means "action." It suggests that we are locked into an action nexus in which the totality of preceding psychological (moral) conditions determine subsequent psychological *and* physical events.

This belief is associated with the understanding that life is a school in which we have to learn a very important lesson, namely, that we determine our future by our present behavior and thoughts. The law of karma ensures that, over long periods of time, we are morally purified. This karmic mechanism is completely impartial. We reap as we sow. Thus, life is not merely the short slice of existence that we are presently experiencing, but a rather protracted affair for which we are solely responsible.

The doctrine of reincarnation does away with the alternative religious belief that, in consonance with our good and bad deeds or volitions, we harvest either eternal happiness or eternal torment in the hereafter. Instead, it places human life within a much larger scale of possibilities and responsibilities. It teaches us that there is scope for moral atonement and spiritual growth, which allows us to remold the course of our life over many embodiments.

But, above all, it challenges us to drop out of this universal recycling by realizing the transcendental Reality that abides beyond both death and life. It is important to bear this fact in mind. The goal of the yogins or ascetics is indeed not to create favorable rebirths for themselves, whether in celestial realms or here on earth. They leave such aspirations to the spiritually immature who are happy with substitute realities.

The sages of mythic spirituality aim at nothing less than total escape from the ever-rotating wheel of life and death. They seek to accomplish this by means of the enlightenment experience in the highest state of mystical union, called *nirvikalpa-samadhi* or "transconceptual ecstasy." This elevated state of consciousness effects a melt-down of the false sense of self, which identifies with a particular body-mind. From that moment on, as we learn from the *Yoga-Sutra* (IV.7), the ascetic's actions or volitions are neither black nor white. The reason for this is that they have ceased to postulate an ego and instead identify with the Self.

Only the human psyche initiates actions prompted by egoic motives. Even the noblest motives are colored by the personality. The Self alone transcends both action and motives. By constantly identifying with the Self, the ascetics bypass the personality, and all their actions are said to be purely spontaneous. We will consider this claim in a later chapter.

SALVATION THROUGH WISDOM

The doctrine of re-embodiment has gone through various stages of development. The most primitive versions are rather crudely animistic, while the most sophisticated interpretation can be found in Buddhism. However, it is in Jainism that we encounter the most detailed analysis of the karmic process. According to the Jainas, karma is a kind of material substance that floats about in the universe like cosmic dust. Transcending it is the human Spirit (atman), which is inherently free and eternal but, in the unenlightened being, experiences itself as bound and limited. The karmic substance is attracted by that self-limiting Spirit, which vibrates at a given rate owing to its volitional activity. Because of the bound Spirit's resident passions (*kashaya*), the karma substance sticks to the person. This influx (*asrava*) of karma into the psyche then shapes the person's destiny, affecting his or her perceptions, knowledge, experience, and overall state of existence.

Only in the case of dispassionate individuals, whose psyche is "dry," does the karmic substance fail to cling to them. They are aware of their true identity and are thus free of all karmic influences.

The contact between Spirit and karmic matter is philosophically problematical, because how can the immaterial Spirit interact with a material substance? The same problem, however, bedevils all idealist traditions in India and elsewhere.

In early Buddhism, which rejected the idealist interpretations of its day, the doctrine of karma is given a unique twist. The Buddhist scholastics speak no longer of *punar-janman* (lit. "rebirth") but of *punar-bhava* (lit. "re-becoming"). The difference between these two formulations consists in that the latter excludes the belief in a transmigrating subject. There is for them no individual that persists through all the countless reincarnations. From the Buddhist perspective, it is wrong to speak of a transmigration of souls.

Buddhists explain the continuity between births with the help of the nexus of codependent origination (*pratitya-samutpada*): The new entity originates in dependence on the totality of the antecedent factors of existence. To illustrate this curious connection, the *Milinda-Panha* uses the image of a torch that is used to kindle another.

The driving force in the process of repeated lives is our volitional activity, regardless of whether it is translated into visible action or not. Thus, our mind determines our future. This is in principle also the view maintained by the teachers of Vedanta. It is through our intentions, which are a powerful form of activity, that the wheel of becoming (*bhava-cakra*) is kept in continual motion.

Although our present existence is the result of previous volitional activity, nevertheless karma only determines the essential nature of the next birth. It fixes the mental and psychosomatic factors and also the overall environmental conditions. It does not predetermine the actual activity carried out in the new existence. From this it is clear that the doctrine of rebirth must not be confused with blind determinism. The human will is free, even though its sphere of possible self-expression is more or less restricted.

The authorities of Vedanta compare the human being to a spider that day in day out weaves itself more and more into its web, until it is completely enveloped by it. The moral of the story is that actions can never lead to the light; they merely enmesh us ever more in matter. Hence Shankara's admonition to all worldlings that they must discontinue their senseless activity and abandon their false hope of finding true happiness in the world. In the first verse of the *Moha-Mudgara* ("Cudgel of Delusion"), one of his popular poems, Shankara pleads:

> O fool!
> Renounce your desire
> to accumulate riches.
> Create in your mind
> pure thoughts, devoid of craving.
> Content your heart with
> what falls to you
> as a gift from past deeds.

In his manual *Upadesha-Sahasri* ("Thousand Teachings"), Shankara outlines the fateful consequences of karma thus:

> The deeds [of past existences] produce the link [of the psyche] with the [new] body. From this connection with the body [come] pleasure and pain. This is followed by attachment and aversion. Thence [follow more] deeds, which result in virtue (*dharma*) or vice (*adharma*). Subsequently the unenlightened [suffers] renewed connection with a body. Thus the world rolls on eternally like a wheel. (II.I.3–4)

Our worldly activity leaves behind traces in the depths of our psyche. These subliminal forces, which are called "activators" (*samskara*), are the real causes of the succession of births and deaths. As long as they are present, the rebirth series cannot come to a standstill. They ignite volitional activity which, in turn, enriches the stock of subliminal activators. This chain can be interrupted at one link only. Neither self-annihilation through suicide (which only involves the physical frame) nor the abstention from volition (which is practically impossible) is the answer. The only way to suspend this cycle is by eradicating the existing stock of activators and preventing the accumulation of new activators, which can be accomplished through the dawning of true gnosis.

STOPPING THE WHEEL OF BECOMING

The elimination of the karmic traces in the subconscious is achieved through a profound inner reorientation or spiritual conversion. Christian theologians employ the Greek term *metanoia* for this reversal. It involves the whole person, manifesting in our thoughts and emotions as well as our actions. This most comprehensive process, which neutralizes the old Adam, calls for systematic discipline over a long period of time.

The Buddha's "noble eightfold path" exemplifies what this entails. It comprises the following eight steps:

1. right vision (*samyag-drishti*), which consists essentially in realizing the transient nature of conditioned existence;

2. right resolve (*samyak-samkalpa*), which is the threefold decision to renounce the impermanent, to practice benevolence, and to abstain from deliberately hurting other beings;

3. right speech (*samyag-vaca*), which consists in guarding one's language;

4. right behavior (*samyak-karmanta*), which is moral conduct, especially the cultivation of the virtues of nonharming, nonstealing, and chastity;

5. right livelihood (*samyag-ajiva*), which refers to the duty of the lay Buddhist to follow a profession in which other beings do not come to harm;

6. right exertion (*samyag-vyayama*), which is the continual effort to prevent unwholesome mental activity and to cultivate wholesome volitions, particularly by guarding the senses;

7. right mindfulness (*samyak-smriti*), which is the effort to make conscious the various somatic and mental processes, especially through the exercise of mindful concentration on otherwise semiconscious or unconscious processes such as breathing;

8. right unification (*samyak-samadhi*), which consists in techniques aimed at the progressive introversion and subsequent dismantling of consciousness, including higher ecstatic or mystical states.

As in the case of the eightfold path of Patanjali, these eight components of the Buddha's "middle way" are not strictly stages forming part of a ladder to liberation. With the exception of the eighth component, which is for advanced practitioners, these practices must be cultivated simultaneously.

Through the complete inner reversal made possible by the various techniques and attitudes recommended by the Buddha and subsequent masters, the production of new unwholesome volition is prevented. Moreover, in the higher stages of mystical experience, the piled-up stock of subliminal activators is consumed by the fire of gnosis.

In Patanjali's Classical Yoga this process is explained in the *klesha* theory. The term *klesha*, which is derived from the verbal root *klish* ("to torment"), is best translated as "cause of suffering." Patanjali distinguished five such causes of suffering. In keeping with the Buddha's vision, he regarded spiritual ignorance (*avidya*) as the primary source of all sorrow. It is the nutrient soil of all other causes of suffering, namely: "I-am-ness" (*asmita*), attachment (*raga*), aversion (*dvesha*), and clinging to life (*abhinivesha*). These instigators of suffering occur in four forms. They are either latent, attenuated, temporarily suppressed, or fully operative.

The interim goal of the yogins is to "thin out," or sublimate, these factors. The next step is to eliminate them completely and even render their future occurrence impossible. When spiritual nescience and its lethal products are fully removed, the adepts gain the highest gnosis, which once and for all transports them out of the sorrowful ocean of conditioned existence. This supreme gnostic realization empowers the adepts to accurately perceive the all-important distinction between the most refined aspect of the human psyche, which is called *sattva* (literally "being-ness"), and the transcendental Self.

The sattva aspect *resembles* the Self in translucency, and so it can easily be confused with the Self by those adepts who are impatient and lacking in discrimination. However, only the realization of the transcendental Spirit, the purusha, brings liberation. For the sattva belongs entirely to the realm of insentient Nature, in which the ever-free Self mysteriously deems itself enmeshed.

Thus, while the experience of the sattva in elevated mystical states is positive and even blissful, it falls short of liberation. Hence it contains an element of suffering, since any experience, even the most sublime, is limited and inevitably comes to an end. Only the realization of the Self, the ultimate Witness, is untainted by space and time and suffering. In the words of the *Bhagavad-Gita* (XIII.31), "this immutable supreme Self is beginningless and beyond the constituents [of Nature]." It is pure luminosity, and no shadow can fall upon it.

The mystical experience of the sattva essence must itself be transcended through gnosis. According to the *Yoga-Sutra* (II.27), the highest form of gnosis yields a sevenfold recognition. The author of the *Yoga-Bhashya* explains that this spontaneous knowledge entails the certainty that the causes of suffering have been completely eliminated. Then the Self abides in its flawless purity, and the cycle of births and deaths is once and for all interrupted.

NOTES

1. For a good coverage of reincarnation beliefs around the world, see J. Head and S.L. Cranson, eds., *Reincarnation: An East-West Anthology* (New York: Crown, 1961). See also W.D. O'Flaherty, ed., *Karma and Rebirth in Classical Indian Traditions* (Berkeley: University of California Press, 1980) and R.W. Neufeldt, ed., *Karma and Rebirth: Post Classical Developments* (New York: SUNY Press, 1986).

2. Not all scholars accept the theory that the Vedic Aryans hailed from the steppes of southern Russia. Some think that the Vedic tribes were indigenous to India and were possibly the builders of the Indus civilization. See, e.g., D. Frawley, *Gods, Sages and Kings: Vedic Secrets of Ancient Civilization* (Salt Lake City, UT: Passage Press, 1991).

CHAPTER 6

THE ASCETIC FLIGHT FROM TIME

TIME, THE OMNIVOROUS DEMON

Perhaps one of the most important characteristics of the mythic consciousness is its rejection of historical or secular time and its tenacious orientation toward the timeless primordial Reality. The mythic consciousness experiences temporality as the root cause of all fears and sorrows. Time is seen as the frustrator of all human hopes. It gnaws away at life itself. As Prince Rama puts it in the *Yoga-Vasishtha* (I.23.3ff.):

Time is like a mouse that completely gnaws through the threads of delicate, hapless thoughts entertained [by people] here [in this world]. (3)

There is nothing here [on earth] that all-voracious Time does not devour. It [swallows] the created world, just as the submarine fire [consumes] the overflowing ocean [at the end of a cosmic cycle]. (4)

Time is the great lord who is equally terrible to all, and [ever] ready to make morsels out of all visible [i.e., manifest] beings. (5)

[Time] is the foundation of all cruelty and greed as well as of all misfortune and unbearable instability. (20)

At the end of a great age (*maha-kalpa*), [Time] plucks the host of gods and antigods (*asura*) like ripe fruit from a tree. (26)

[Time] destroys [the beauty of] youth, as the moon does the lotus [at night]. [It ravishes] life, as the lion does the elephant. There is nothing, however significant or insignificant, that this thief does not steal. (42)

Although time is infinitely creative, it is nonetheless incessantly engaged in the destruction of all things. The Sanskrit word for time is *kala*, which means "black" and "death." This color symbolism makes the point that time is the opposite of Reality, which is characteristically associated with white brilliance—the supernal light that is seen at the moment of death.

The *Yoga-Vasishtha* (VI.7.34) compares time to a potter who, continually turning his wheel, produces innumerable pots only to smash them whenever he fancies doing so. This simile suggests the popular metaphor of the "wheel of time" (*kala-cakra*). This metaphor goes back to the era of the *Rig-Veda*. In one hymn (I.164.11), the blind seer Dirghatamas poses a riddle when he says that "around the heaven revolves the ever-unaging twelve-spoked wheel of order (*rita*)." We can see in this a reference to the zodiacal belt, the cosmic engine that is thought to determine all life on earth.

In another verse of the same hymn, 360 spokes—the 360 degrees of the sun's movement through the zodiac, roughly corresponding to the days of the year—are mentioned. These are said to turn unfailingly, without deviation. The wheel of time is pulled by the brilliant steed, which is the sun. The sun has anciently been recognized as the prime life-giving force of the world, a powerful connecting link between the physical reality and the divine dimension. The sun is linked with time and death as well as the timeless and immortal Being. It is a principal factor in maintaining the cosmic order (rita).

Time tears asunder the original wholeness, thus depriving all beings of their true identity. They drift powerlessly in the ocean of time, now on the surface (during life), now beneath it (after death). Not even the celestial beings are safe. In the words of the *Mahabharata* epic (XI.2.8 and 24):

Time pulls along all creatures, even the gods. There is none dear to Time, none hateful.

Time cooks [all] beings. Time destroys [all] creatures. [When everything else is] asleep, time is awake. Time is hard to overcome.

The *Shiva-Purana* (VII.1.7), an encyclopedic work from the medieval period, contains a eulogy on the grandeur of Time. The following is a summary of this section: Everything originates from time and is annihilated by it. The universe whirls on, propelled by time's creativity and destructiveness. Time unites and separates creatures. It cannot be bribed or thwarted. There is no escape from time merely by means of intellectual effort, or by restraining the senses, or even by imbibing rejuvenating elixirs. Inscrutable Time overwhelms and controls all through the law of karma. Only God Shiva, the Ultimate, is outside the dominion of time. Indeed, he is the master of time. It is through the agency of time that Shiva rules supreme in the world.

This echoes an ancient tradition, which more than a thousand years before the composition of the *Shiva-Purana* was given expression in the *Bhagavad-Gita* (X.33–34). Here Lord Krishna, a full incarnation of the Divine, says of himself:

. . . I am imperishable Time. I am the Supporter facing everywhere.

I am also all-seizing death, and the origin of what is to be . . .

Hence when the spiritual adept identifies with and actually *becomes* the Divine, he or she likewise conquers time.

MYTHIC TIME AND THE TIMELESS

Although the mythic consciousness possesses an acute awareness of time, its time experience differs profoundly from that of the mental consciousness. For, as Jean Gebser explained, in the mythic structure of consciousness people's awareness of space is as yet dormant. Hence their sense of time is also not yet spatialized. Temporal linearity—the "arrow of time"—is the discovery of the mental structure of consciousness.

Mythic time is circular or cyclic movement: from aeon to aeon, from spring to winter, from new moon to new moon, from birth to death. In China this universal periodicity is fittingly symbolized by a dragon biting its own tail. Indian mythology depicts time as the giant bird Garuda, Vishnu's mount. Garuda is said to feed upon innumerable serpents, which represent the cycles within cycles.

Mythic time is the recurrent flow of events, as it is so aptly captured in the Sanskrit term *samsara*. This word, which refers to the universe, is derived from the verbal root *sri* ("to flow, glide"). Thus, samsara is that which flows on uninterruptedly only to turn back upon itself. It is the cycle of existence in which all creatures are trapped as in a grinding mill.

The mythic consciousness operates in the field of polarities, rather than dual opposites. Its time sense is based on movement, but a movement that is still prespatial. It is oblivious to perspectivity. The mythic spatial sense is similar to the experience of space in our dreams. The peculiar landscapes of our dreams are not sharply three-dimensional. They have an aspatial quality that is coextensive with the activities of our dreaming psyche. The mythic space can be described as two-dimensional, undulating always between two poles.

This circular picture of life was shattered only with the emergence of the directional thinking characteristic of the mental structure of consciousness. It gave birth to the experience of space and time as two distinct and even contrary phenomena.

THE TRANSCENDENCE OF TIME

The attitude of the inmate of the mythic structure of consciousness toward time is one of discontent, nonacceptance, and therefore designed neglect. This is borne out by the mythic search for primordial Time, which is really the Timeless.

In the *Maitri-Upanishad* (VI.15), we find quoted an ancient stanza, which asks: "It is Time that cooks created things. . . . In what, however, is Time cooked?" The verse continues to say that those who know the answer do indeed know the sacred tradition, the *Vedas*. The riddle's solution is that time resides in the Timeless. That Timeless is the true fulfillment of human existence. This is a fundamental credo of all spiritual schools. According to the *Maitri-Upanishad* (VI.15), Reality is comprised of two levels:

There are two forms of *brahman*: time and the Timeless. That which is prior to the sun is the Timeless (*akala*), the Impartite, whereas that which begins with the sun is time, which is partitioned. Verily, the form of that which is partitioned is the year. From the year, in truth, [all] creatures are

produced. Verily, through the year, after having been produced, they grow. In the year, they disappear. Therefore the
year, verily, is Prajapati [the Creator], is time, is food, is the
abode of the Absolute (*brahman*), is the Self.

The same scripture contains this important practical clue:
"Whoever reverences time as the Absolute, from him time recoils."
The path of Yoga is such reverencing, and thus it is a way out of
time. "The yogin [who is] yoked through ecstasy . . . is not de-
voured by time," declares the author of the *Hatha-Yoga-Pradipika*
(IV.108) confidently. Similar statements can be found scattered
throughout the vast mass of India's liberation literature.

The perfected adept is also referred to as "one who has transcended time" (*kala-atita*). This Sanskrit designation corresponds
to the more frequent expression *guna-atita* or "one who has transcended the constituents [of Nature]." Primordial Time is *nirguna*,
that is, beyond the scope of the three types of constituents (*guna*)
that compose conditioned existence. It is also said to be
"impartite" (*akala*), which is to say, it is eternal present. It is in the
Timeless that the adepts see their ultimate salvation.

To be sure, the mythic penchant for the Timeless is still alive in
us today. We would expect this to be so, given the fact that we are
the sum total of all structures of consciousness. As the renowned
historian of religion Mircea Eliade observed, we moderns have our
own peculiar way of avoiding time and seeking immersion into
the Timeless. He wrote:

> The defence against Time which is revealed to us in every
> kind of mythological attitude but which is, in fact, inseparable
> from the human condition, reappears variously disguised in
> the modern world, but above all in its distractions, its amuse-
> ments.[1]

Thus, our pursuit of ephemeral pleasurable goals forms a Yoga
of sorts, because we are fairly singleminded about it. However, the
modern substitute quest lacks the benefits of a genuine sacred
path. While it may fill us temporarily, it cannot ultimately fulfill us.

Those on whom time weighs heavily suffer from ennui, or
cosmic boredom and meaninglessness. This is not a mood that we

can easily endure, and so we become addicted to new experiences. In fact, we are brought up to cram as many experiences as possible into the short "space" of a single lifetime. This represents our attempt to drown the thunderous silence that arises from the Infinite when the mind is in idle motion. It is an abortive attempt, to be sure. For the Timeless cannot be wished away. It will always be present in the midst of our time-bound experiences.

If we moderns are afraid of the sacred, it is because we have become alienated from it. We are afraid of the depths of our own psyche, where time stands still. The sages of modern India look in astonishment at our feeble attempts to control the flux of time by cultivating ever new experiences and sensations. They have understood that the only way to conquer time is by perfectly transcending it, by discovering our original roots in the Timeless.

NOTE

1. M. Eliade, *Myths, Dreams and Mysteries* (London: Fontana Library, 1968), p. 36.

CHAPTER 7

THE ALCHEMY OF RENUNCIATION

LETTING GO OF CONVENTIONAL LIFE

When the world is viewed merely as a seat of sorrow and adversity, there is ultimately no other choice than to step out of it. In other words, we must renounce and abandon everything that the universe harbors in its infinite circumference. For the mythic consciousness, renunciation is the only road to salvation. As the *Mahanarayana-Upanishad* (XII.14a) declares:

> Not through work, not through progeny, and not through wealth but by renunciation have some attained immortality.

Only singleminded devotion to the transcendental Being promises the end of all suffering. Everything else merely drags us closer to the mill-wheel of the world. "Man is formed of desire," declared Sage Yajnavalkya, quoting an ancient stanza. He explained:

> As is his desire, so is his will; as is his will, so proves his deed; as turns out his deed, so he obtains [a wholesome or unwholesome form of existence].[1]

By being intent on the good, we not only improve our present life but attain to a good incarnation in the future. However, if we are preeminently motivated by evil intentions, our present life as well as our future embodiment will be afflicted with great difficulties. In contrast to these two types of destiny, the ascetics who have disengaged themselves from all desire and solely aspire to the realization of the Self transcend good and evil. For them, life begins at death. In their case, death is truly a birth, because upon dropping the body they consciously enter the supreme Being.

The famous Indian poet Bartrihari, who died in 651 A.D., is said to have renounced the life of fame and debauchery that he led at the royal court of his brother Vikramaditya of Ujjayini in order to dedicate himself wholeheartedly to the quest for liberation. His *Vairagya-Shataka* ("Century on Renunciation"), which was apparently composed shortly after his change of mind, is a document of deep human value. Two verses are particularly stirring:

Enjoyments are never enjoyed, but we ourselves are enjoyed. Asceticism is never kindled, but we ourselves are burnt up. Time does not pass, but we pass. Our thirsts are never quenched, but we ourselves are consumed. (verse 7)

In enjoyment lies the fear of disease; in social status, the fear of loss; in wealth, the fear of the king; in honor, the fear of humiliation; in strength, the fear of the opponent; in beauty, the fear of old age; in erudition, the fear of the disputant; in virtue, the fear of the seducer; in the body, the fear of death. All the things of this world, pertaining to a person, are attended with fear. Renunciation alone grants a person fearlessness. (verse 31)

Fear arises through each contact with the world. Hence to the mythic consciousness, which does not know or count on the inner type of renunciation, the only possible answer is to conquer fear by withdrawing from all mundane objects. Renunciation, in other words, is the path into homelessness, into the seclusion of forests, deserts, or mountain caves, to the no-man's-land outside conventional society.

What this means is vividly described in the *Markandeya-Purana* (XXI.4ff.), where the sage Dattatreya instructs his disciple Alarka about the strict, almost ritualistic life of the ascetic:

He should set his foot only after [the path] has been purified by the eye; he should drink only water filtered through cloth; only utter words purified by truth, and only think of what has been purified throughout by the wisdom-faculty (*buddhi*).

The knower of Yoga should nowhere be a guest, and he should not participate in ancestor worship, sacrifices, pilgrimages to [the shrines of] gods and festivities; he also should not mix with the crowd for purposes of demonstration.

The knower of Yoga should wander about begging [his daily

food] and live off what he finds in the refuse, at places where no smoke arises [from the hearth], where the coal is extinguished, among all those who have already eaten, but also not continually among these three.

Since the crowd despises and mocks him because of this, the *yogin* should, yoked [in Yoga], tread the path of the good, [in order that he might] not be tarnished.

He should seek alms among the householders and the huts of mendicant monks: their mode of life is considered the foremost and best.

The ascetic (*yati*) should furthermore also always stay among the pious, self-controlled and magnanimous householders versed in the Veda.

In addition of course [he should stay] among the innocent and those who are not outcastes. Begging among the casteless is the lowest mode of life which he could wish.

The begged food [may consist of] gruel, diluted buttermilk or milk, barley broth, fruit, roots, millet, corn, oil-cake, or groats.

And these are pleasant eatables which support the *yogins'* [striving after] perfection (*siddhi*). The sage should turn to them with devotedness and highest concentration (*samadhi*).

After first having drunk water, he should collect himself silently. Then he should [offer] the first oblation to the [vital force] called *prana*.

The second [oblation] should be to *apana*, the next to *samana*, the fourth to *udana* and the fifth to *vyana*.

After having completed one oblation after the other, [all the while practicing] the restraint of the vital force, he may then enjoy the remainder to his heart's content. Taking again water and rinsing, he should touch his heart.

Nonstealing, chastity, dispassion, absence of greed, and nonharming are the five most important vows of the mendicant.

Absence of wrath, obedience to the teacher, purity, moderation in eating, sustained study—these are the five well-known restraints (*niyama*).

Above all, [the *yogin*] should dedicate himself to knowledge that leads to the goal. The multiplicity of knowledge as it exists here [on earth] is an obstacle in Yoga.

He who seized by thirst dashes along [in the belief that he must] know this or that, will not even in a thousand aeons obtain that which is to be known [viz., the ultimate Reality].

Abandoning society, curbing wrath, eating moderately, and controlling the senses, he should block the [nine] gates [of the body] by means of the wisdom-faculty (buddhi) and let the mind come to rest in meditation.

That *yogin* who is yoked incessantly should continually practice meditation in empty rooms, caves, and in the forest.

Control of speech, control of activity, and control of the mind—these are the three [masteries]. He who [practices] these restraints unfailingly, [is called] a great "three restraints" ascetic.

Who, O king, is dear or not dear to him for whom everything consists of the Self: that which is real and unreal in the world, the good and the bad?

Whose wisdom-faculty is purified, for whom gold or a lump of earth are the same and who thus, same-minded toward all beings, realizes the supreme State, the eternally undecaying Transcendent—he is not born again.

Excellent are the Vedas and all sacrifices. [Better] than sacrifice is recitation, and the path of knowledge [is even better] than recitation. [More excellent] than knowledge is meditation that is devoid of desire for any contact [with sense objects]. When this is accomplished, the Eternal is won.

He who is collected, absorbed in the Absolute, attentive, pure, and in extreme rapture (*rati*) and of controlled senses—that great soul (*maha-atman*) may obtain this Yoga; subsequently he is sure to gain liberation.

RADICAL ABANDONMENT OF THE EGO
AND THE UNIVERSE

In mythic spirituality, the break with the world is radical and abrupt. One has either seceded once and for all from its deceptive pleasures and adopted the austere life of an ascetic, or one nourishes a greedy lust in the bustle of mundane life. There is no position of compromise. It is either God or the world, Truth or falsehood, Bliss or sorrow, the Eternal or ruin. This attitude is beautifully illustrated in a parable told by Ramakrishna, one of the great sages of nineteenth century India:

A woman once addressed her husband thus: "Dear, I am worried about my brother. These last months he has toyed with the idea of adopting the life of a renunciate. And he tries to reduce his needs bit by bit." — "You need not be anxious about your brother," her husband replied. "He will never become a renunciate, because that is not the way to do it." The woman asked: "How then does one become a renunciate?" The husband replied: "Behold! Thus." And he tore his garment, took two pieces and wrapped them around his loins. Explaining to his wife that from now on he would regard her and all other women as mothers, he turned around and left his home for good.[2]

Renunciation ultimately means fearlessness, for when one has left behind everything there can be no more fear of loss. What the unenlightened individual fears the most is to lose his or her ego-identity. When renunciation is radically true, the sense of self is abandoned together with all the countless objects of the cosmos. Perfect world- and self-negation are marks of Self-realization. Fear is only possible where two or more things coexist. Since the Self is singular, its realization coincides with the eradication of the deep-seated fear of death.

For us Westerners this readiness for total renunciation is startling and disturbing. Our psychic life is relatively impoverished, and we live almost exclusively on the surface of the psyche, with our energies dedicated to the external world. The craving for sensations appears to us as the norm.

In contrast, the ascetics who are anchored in the mythic structure of consciousness view the centrifugal, object-centered attitude of the Western mind as spiritually deficient. They regard it as the product of a profound metaphysical ignorance, which occludes the transcendental Reality. It is an orientation riddled with self-delusion and illusion (maya).

In the same way that greed for experiences and self-survival ensnares unenlightened individuals in suffering, the disposition of thirstlessness effects their liberation. Radical renunciation extends over the whole universe in all its many layers and countless forms of manifestation. Even the "inner" realms, or celestial spheres, are included in this act, since they too are impermanent and not conducive to true happiness and freedom.

True renunciation mobilizes forces within the human psyche that can work miracles of spiritual transformation. While the various practices of unification serve the agglomeration of psychic power, renunciation establishes the inner vacuum that is necessary for the proper utilization of the accumulated psychic energy.

Thus it becomes clear why both poles of the spiritual path stand in need of simultaneous cultivation. Both the blocking-out of multiplicity and the actual process of unification are interdependent aspects of the alchemical process that leads to a person's spiritual rebirth, the new Adam. When the unification pole is preponderant, there is a strong likelihood of the misdirection of the accumulated psychic energy, possibly leading to inflation and power mongering. When the renunciation pole prevails, the likely consequence will be acute introversion without proper channeling of the stored energy, which may cause a breakdown of the ascetic's physical and mental health. As the *Bhagavad-Gita* (II.48) emphasizes, Yoga is "equanimity" (*samatva*)—a hair-trigger balance that needs to be maintained in all aspects of the path to the transcendental Singularity.

NOTES

1. *Brihad-Aranyaka-Upanishad* IV.4.6.

2. E. von Pelet, ed., *Worte des Ramakrishna* (Erlenbach/Zurich, 1930), p. 79. Translated from the German by the present author.

CHAPTER 8

DISMANTLING THE EGO-PERSONALITY

THE EGO AS ENEMY

Spiritual life can be viewed from a variety of standpoints: that of purification, unification, liberation from the bonds of karma, the eradication of suffering, and not least the progressive dismantling of the finite personality. All these viewpoints are equally valuable and useful, as they disclose different aspects of the great process of spiritual transmutation.

Profane individuals are full of themselves. They do not know the creative Void, the pause between breaths, which alone secures their salvation. As the anonymous author of the *Theologia Germanica* (III), a fourteenth-century German work, observed: The fall of Adam did not come about because he ate of the forbidden apple, but solely because of his fixed attachment to the "I," "Me," and "Mine."

It is, the mystical writer continued, the self-will that burns in hell for the purification of the soul. Hardened egocentricity alone is the reason why humans are cast into the whirling wheel of existence. For it is the prism of the ego that fragments the single Being so that it appears as multiple subjects and objects. It breaks, as it were, the uniform "white light" of the Self into the countless colors of the spectrum. It occludes the Spirit, thereby causing untold suffering and unhappiness.

For this reason the only road to salvation lies in the radical rejection and ultimate uprooting of the ego-personality. This negation of the ego is characteristic of the mythic striving for unification. Over and over, the sacred scriptures condemn the ego, which is held responsible for our distortion of reality.

The ego is portrayed as the arch fiend of the Spirit. It divides where there is essentially only oneness and thus creates existential tension grounded in fear. As Shankara puts it in verse 303 of his *Viveka-Cudamani* ("Crest-Jewel of Discrimination"), the ego is to the human psyche as poison is to the body. In verse 300, he compares the ego with Rahu, the ascending lunar node. According to mythology, Rahu devours the full moon, which represents the Self.

Like a three-headed serpent monster, the ego bars the way to the hidden treasure within us. The ego is triple-headed, because its existence is due to the interaction of the three primary constituents of the created universe.

THE PLACE OF THE EGO IN THE COSMIC HIERARCHY

The doctrine of the three *gunas* counts among the most original contributions of the ancient Samkhya-Yoga tradition. This theory seems to have been known already at the time of the older *Upanishads*, yet surprisingly enough it was not until the sixteenth century that it was given a more elaborate philosophical treatment.[1] These gunas are thought to be the ultimate building blocks of phenomenal reality, the irreducible "particles" of Nature. Infinite in number, they show a triple mode of functioning:

1. *sattva* (lit. "beingness"), which is the aspect of translucency or purity;

2. *rajas* (from the verbal root *raj/ranj*, meaning "to be brilliant"), which is the quality of dynamism;

3. *tamas* (from the verbal root *tam*, meaning "to languish"), which is the principle of inertia.

Ishvara Krishna, the founder of Classical Samkhya, defines these three modal functions of Nature as follows:

The constituents are of the nature of pleasantness, unpleasantness, and oppression and have the purpose of illumination, activity, and obscuration [respectively]; they dominate each other, are mutually dependent, productive, and co-operative in their movements.—*Sattva* is regarded as buoyant and illuminating, *rajas* as exciting and mobile, and *tamas* as heavy and concealing. Their activity is purposive, similar to a lamp, [which consists of diverse components, like wick, oil and fire, whose harmonious interaction produces a single phenomenon, viz. light].[2]

The combined activity of the gunas produces the cosmos in its entirety. In the transcendental matrix of the world, out of which evolve in hierarchic sequence the multiple levels and objects of existence, these primary constituents are in a state of relative balance. The disturbance of this original equilibrium initiates the cosmogenesis, or emergence of the universe.

The first evolute to appear out of the unmanifest core of the world is buddhi, which is generic being-consciousness. It has a preponderance of sattva. Out of this nonmaterial soup crystallizes, under the impact of rajas, the ontic principle of individuation, which is widely called *ahamkara* ("I-maker").

The I-maker, in turn, is the starting point of a bifurcated development, caused by a prevalence of tamas. On the one side, the eleven senses (including the lower mind) evolve from it. On the other side, it gives rise to the five types of supermatter (*tanmatra*) and, by way of further condensation, to their corresponding material elements.

In other words, the world-ground gives birth to all material as well as psychic phenomena. The question of what caused the initial disturbance, which led from pure potentiality to the actual manifestation of the world, is answered by Yoga and Samkhya in a philosophically rather unsatisfactory manner. According to the former system, it is the will of the Lord (*ishvara*) that inaugurates the process; for the latter tradition, it is the influence of the still unemancipated Self-monads (*purusha*) which clamor for experience.

This short discussion of the gunas was necessary in order to form a more precise idea of the ontological position of the ego within the Samkhya-Yoga scheme. As stated above, the first principle to evolve from the undifferentiated potentiality field of Nature is buddhi. It is the mediator between the unmanifest world-ground and the universe of differentiated phenomena, both visible and invisible.

The buddhi contains in germ all material and psychic realities that could ever take form on any of the levels of existence. At the ontic level of the buddhi, subjectivity and objectivity are still merged. It is a homogeneous field, which serves as the medium of the lower types of yogic ecstasy in which a relative coincidence of subject and object is experienced.

The buddhi resembles the structure-giving *logos* of the Greek philosophers, but we may also characterize it as a generic consciousness, because it stores all subliminal impressions, which drive the destiny of every being.

The transition from uniformity to multiplicity takes place on the level of the I-maker. It is the direct source of the individualized or lower mind (*manas*), the five cognitive and the five conative senses, as well as the five correlated elements together with their subtle counterparts (sound, sight, and so on). We can readily appreciate why in the yogic program of involution the I-maker, or ego, must be eliminated at any cost. It is the only real barrier on the path of unification. It blocks our conscious access to the subject-object identity on the level of buddhi and beyond.

DECONSTRUCTING THE HUMAN PERSONALITY

The reason for the scrupulous excision of the ego, strived for in the schools of mythic spirituality, is that this will lead to a supra-egoic consciousness (buddhi) and, ultimately, even to the realization of the transcendental Awareness, or Self. This procedure can be explained in terms of a process of progressive de-personalization. Meister Eckhart, the great German mystic and scholastic of the European Middle Ages, used an even stronger expression. He spoke of the need for a complete "de-humanization." As he put it:

> As long as we are human and as long as there is anything human in us, and we are in motion, we are unable to behold God.[3]

It is clear from this that Eckhart did not mean dehumanization in the sense of becoming brutish. Rather, he intended it to suggest our divinization—a way of putting it that would not have been permissible at his time.

The underlying idea of this process of de-humanization, or (to coin a term) transhumanization, is quite simple: In order to realize our true Identity, which is the Spirit, we must drop everything that makes us creatures rather than the Creator. The Spirit is neither male nor female, old nor young, rich nor poor, esteemed nor despised. All such human parameters do not apply to it.

If we want to realize the Spirit, or Self, we must transcend our

typically human characteristics by which we tend to define ourselves. This is accomplished through spiritual discipline, which is
essentially an effort to deconstruct ourselves. Through such practices as meditation and renunciation, the ascetics seek to unravel
the web of human complexities. The caterpillar becomes a butter-
fly only by breaking out of the cocoon. Humans become the Spirit
only by dismantling the encrusted personality, which is fixed on
the unenlightened ego.

This process of deconstruction appears to be basic to any spiritual system, although it may be formulated in many different
ways. Shankara, for example, put it thus in his *Nirvana-Shatka*
("The Six on Extinction"):

> I am not intuition nor reason,
> not I-maker nor experience.
> Neither hearing am I, nor speech;
> not smell nor sight.
> Earth and ether,
> fire and air
> I am not.
> I am Shiva,
> in form of awareness and bliss.
> Shiva am I.
>
> I am not the sentient life-force;
> and nor am I the five wind-currents.
> I am not the seven parts
> nor the five sheaths;
> not mouth, nor hand, nor foot.
> Genitalia nor anus
> I am not.
> I am Shiva . . .
>
> To me belong not hate nor passion,
> not greed nor power of delusion,
> not gaiety nor dissatisfaction,
> nor Becoming.

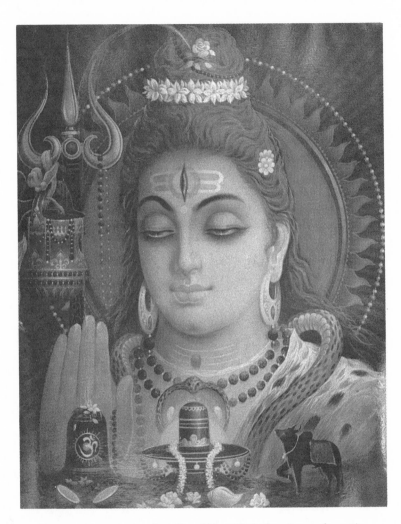

*Contemporary poster depicting Shiva, God of yogins and ascetics,
in a meditative mood, with his right hand raised in blessing.*

I am without law and aim,
without craving and salvation.
I am Shiva . . .

I know not of good and evil,
naught of happiness and pain,
nor of mantra nor the altar,
nor of sacrifice and Vedas.
I am neither the enjoyer
nor the food to be enjoyed,
Nor am I enjoying itself.
I am Shiva . . .

To me belong not death nor fear,
I am beyond the rule of caste;
without parents do I stand,
and I am even without birth.
Without relatives and friends,
without teacher and pupil I am.
I am Shiva . . .

I am changeless—shape amorphous;
omnipresent I remain,
standing still beyond the senses.
I am without deliverance.
Neither am I tangible.
I am Shiva,
in form of awareness and bliss.
Shiva am I.

The same idea is expressed differently in a legend found in the *Mahabharata* (IX.38.38ff.), which serves well to conclude this chapter. The ascetic Mankanaka happened to cut himself on a sharp blade of *kusha* grass and to his utter delight discovered that it was not blood that flowed from the wound, but plant juice: a sure token of his spiritual accomplishment. He burst out in a wild, unbridled dance, which was so fierce that it threatened to upset the balance of the whole earth. Concerned about what might happen, the sages decided to approach Shiva, the supreme Lord of the universe, and ask him to put an end to Mankanaka's frenzy.

Instantly grasping the full significance of the situation, Shiva assumed a human body and appeared before the wildly excited ascetic. Mankanaka promptly exploded into rigmarole about his unparalleled achievement. Shiva intimated to him that he was not in the least impressed. Then he cut his own finger tip, and from the wound welled white ash.

Mankanaka was instantly brought to his senses. Throwing himself at Lord Shiva's feet, he humbly begged for forgiveness. The white ash symbolizes, of course, Shiva's total and irrevocable dispassion and his perfect transcendence of phenomenal existence.

The ascetic Mankanaka had surpassed the ordinary human condition. His veins carried vegetable juice instead of blood. But he had not entirely transcended it, for pride of achievement held him back from the ultimate realization. Lord Shiva reminded him that even the slightest trace of egoity must be eradicated in order to realize God. The ego-personality must be burned to ash. Only then will true freedom and bliss manifest.

NOTES

1. See the *Yoga-Varttika* of Vijnana Bhikshu, which is a detailed exposition of Patanjali's *Yoga-Sutra*.

2. *Samkhya-Karika*, verses 12 and 13. See also *Yoga-Bhashya* II.18.

3. J. Quint, ed., *Meister Eckehart: Deutsche Predigten und Traktate* (Munich: Carl Hanser Verlag, 1955), p. 402. The quote is from sermon 53. The English rendering is by the present author.

CHAPTER 9

THE CRISIS OF INNER AWAKENING

THE TURNING-POINT

The urge for transcendence is an integral part of human life. Depending on the individual's psychological make-up and native spiritual maturity, this urge can announce itself as either a vague existential anxiety, an indefinable religious yearning, or a sudden full-blown passion for the divine. When we become conscious of this urge in us, it inevitably provokes a crisis.

A classic example of this is Prince Arjuna, whose heroism is recounted in the *Mahabharata* epic. His hour of spiritual reckoning is told in the *Bhagavad-Gita*, which forms part of that great epic. Arjuna and his army were facing the enemy on the battlefield. Suddenly, the prince realized that he was about to slaughter relatives, teachers, and friends. He was overcome by great confusion and despair.

Down-hearted, he cast away his bow and arrows. All at once, everything seemed to be called into question. Arjuna had awakened to the utter transiency and ferocity of life.[1] Philosopher and statesman Sarvepalli Radhakrishnan articulated this moment as follows:

> For every individual there comes an hour sometime or other, for nature is not in a hurry, when everything that he can do for himself fails, when he sinks into the gulf of utter blackness, an hour when he would give all that he has for one gleam of light, for one sign of the divine.[2]

Another classic example of such a spiritual awakening is found in the opening section of the *Katha-Upanishad* ("Secret Doctrine of the Kathas"), a scripture dating back to the fifth century B.C. Here the story of the youthful seeker of truth, Naciketas, is told—a story that was probably current already at the time of the

Rig-Veda, many centuries earlier.[3] The name Naciketas is composed of *na* ("not") and *ciketas* ("perceived"). It refers to the ineffable Reality, which lies beyond the ken of the senses and the mind. Clearly, the name was bestowed on the young man as a form of spiritual empowerment.

Naciketas was indeed spiritually ahead of Arjuna, for he did not hesitate to sacrifice himself in order to gain eternal Life. The brahmin youth witnessed his father giving away all his livestock in honor of the Divine. Since the cows were too old to give either milk or calves, Naciketas thought they made an unworthy gift. He reverently approached his father and asked, "To whom will you give me?" In those days, children were the property of their parents.

Naciketas had to repeat his question twice. Finally, irritated by his son's impertinence, the father replied, "I give you to the Lord of Death!" In modern parlance, this translates into "Go to Hell!" We may understand the father's response as a curse, which took immediate magical effect. Perhaps the boy was instantly struck by illness.

We are told that for three full days Naciketas was in the "house of Death," waiting for Lord Yama to take him to his realm. When the God of Death finally returned, he generously offered the brahmin youth three boons for waiting so patiently.

For his first boon, Naciketas asked that his father should receive him with open arms when he is released from the abode of Death. For his second wish, he asked Lord Yama for instruction in the secret teaching of the fire sacrifice, which leads to the heavenly realm. For his third boon, he chose initiation into the secrets of final liberation. The Lord of Death refused, offering riches and a long life instead.

But the youth stood his ground, and in the end Lord Yama reluctantly consented to instruct him about the cause of rebirth and the path to immortality. Naciketas returned to the world of the living with a wisdom that, we may assume, brought him freedom from death through the realization of the transcendental Self.

In the medieval *Yoga-Vasishtha* (I.3ff.), the spiritual awakening of the Prince Rama of Ayodhya is described in vivid and captivating terms. One day, the fifteen-year-old Rama embarked on a pilgrimage to various sacred sites. On his return, he became increasingly withdrawn. He hardly ate anything and spent his days in solitude and silence. His body grew emaciated and weak.

His father, King Dasharatha, became rather concerned about the prince. When asked what was troubling him, Rama replied that he was not worried about anything. Vashishtha, the illustrious sage and royal adviser, diagnosed Rama's withdrawal immediately, but merely told the king not to be concerned.

It so happened that another mighty sage, Vishvamitra, was visiting the royal court at the time. He had in fact come to claim Rama as his disciple. Not wishing to lose his son, King Dasharatha pleaded with the sage to wait until Rama was older, but Vishvamitra would hear none of it. In the face of Vishvamitra's ire, the ruler had no choice but to summon his son. The chamberlain was sent to fetch him but returned without Rama, saying that the prince was in a state of melancholy abstraction and did not wish to be disturbed.

Vishvamitra recognized at once that the prince's condition had no ordinary causes. He told everyone that Rama was in the throes of a spiritual crisis, provoked not by morose thoughts or dark emotions, but by the intrusion of a higher intelligence. The guards were sent to the prince, but he was already on his way to the throne room where the court was assembled. Rama politely saluted everyone and then offered the following explanation for his peculiar behavior:

> During my pilgrimage, I had a number of insights that profoundly shook my faith in worldly things. In me grew a sense of dispassion that gradually made me want to discard all sensual enjoyments. What good are worldly pleasures? They merely hasten our death, like a hurricane uprooting a whole forest. Are we not born to die, only to be reborn again? The body is just a tangled mass of flesh, bones, and veins, tending to become easily exhausted and to fall ill at the slightest provocation. There is nothing more despicable and pitiable than the body. This propped-up hovel inspires no confidence in me. I do not belong to this body, nor does it belong to me.
>
> There is no permanence in anything. Life is as fickle as a

drop of water on a leaf. Everywhere I perceive vice, decay, and danger. All our possessions are the soil from which springs penury. Objects are detached from one another and independent from the mind. It is only in our imagination that we link them to ourselves. It is the mind that creates the illusion of an objective world.

Of what use is royalty? Who am I? Whence is this universe? All things are but vanities. I am disgusted with the world. The only thought that consumes me like a wild fire is the question of how all this suffering can be alleviated.[4]

Rama's unexpected speech astonished everyone. Then the mighty sage Vishvamitra stepped forward and heaped praise upon the youthful prince for his keen understanding of the nature of existence. Then he and Sage Vashishtha proceeded to instruct him in the finer details of the spiritual path. Rama proved a worthy disciple and, later, became a benevolent and enlightened ruler.

Another prince who underwent a spiritual crisis but who renounced his royalty to become one of India's greatest adepts was Gautama the Buddha. He had been brought up completely sheltered from ordinary life. He was shocked out of his innocence when he first ventured forth from the protective environment of his father's palace.

On his first three outings, the prince encountered upsetting testimonies of the impermanency of life. He saw an old man shaking in all his limbs, a sick person lying on the dirty road, and a corpse. On his fourth and last outing, Gautama caught sight of a mendicant monk standing with peaceful indifference on the roadside, and this picture kindled in him a sudden desire to likewise renounce the world.

Soon after this experience, he left the paternal palace never to return. Henceforth he dedicated himself to a life of austerity, which culminated six years later in his enlightenment at the age of thirty-five.

Also in the sixth century B.C., Prince Vardhamana, who is held to have founded Jainism, renounced his throne to adopt the life of a naked mendicant. Since his youth, he had been an exceptional individual. At the age of thirty, the deities urged him to renounce his householder status. Apparently he was more than ready. According to some traditions, he promptly divested himself of all his garments and pulled out his hair by hand. Twelve years, six months, and fifteen days after taking the vow of renunciation, Vardhamana attained enlightenment. He became a *jina*, one who is victorious over death and destiny. Henceforth the Jainas remembered him as Mahavira, the "great hero."

RIDING THE CURRENT TOWARD FREEDOM

In our lifetime, we all are bound to experience adversity, illness, and death. These experiences fill everyone with anxiety, though only in a few people do they have initiatory force. These are the spiritual seekers, who have become sensitive to the extreme limitation and relativity of human existence. For them, suffering becomes an important turning-point—a threshold to the unitive life. Rather than being merely a frustrating experience, suffering points the spiritually sensitive individual to the transcendental Reality, or Spirit.

When we cross this threshold, our hunger for life is transformed into a deep and lasting yearning for Being. This is the point where, in Christian parlance, the new Adam is conceived. His birth is realized during spiritual initiation, while his death coincides with the realization of the Divine. This process can be depicted in the shape of a spiral.

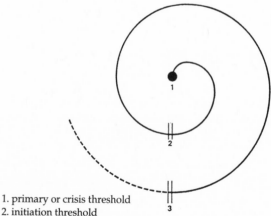

1. primary or crisis threshold
2. initiation threshold
3. realization threshold

A particular feature of the primary threshold of awakening, the initial transformative crisis, is its immanent directedness. As soon as a person has set foot on it, he or she is almost compelled to decide for spiritual rebirth. In this it differs from all other crisis situations of life, which could be regarded as preparations for the great awakening.

In Mahayana Buddhism, this phenomenon is known as the "generation of the will for enlightenment" (*bodhi-citta-utpada*). The Sanskrit term *bodhi-citta* is often rendered as "thought of enlightenment," but *citta* is here more than thought. It is a profound urge that wells up deep within the psyche. It is stronger than all other motivations, and progressively guides the spiritual aspirant to his or her final destination: enlightenment (*bodhi*).

The Buddhist poet and adept Shantideva, who lived in the eighth century A.D., described the generation of this urge for liberation in his own case. In the opening chapter of his celebrated work *Bodhicarya-Avatara* ("Manifestation of the Way to Enlightenment"), Shantideva writes:

> This hard-to-obtain auspicious moment has arrived, leading to the achievement of a person's [ultimate] well-being. If it is not used now, will there ever be another opportunity? (verse 4)

> This will for enlightenment is to be understood as twofold. Briefly, it is the idea of dedication to enlightenment and then the actual pilgrimage toward enlightenment. (verse 15)

> As soon as one resolves to free oneself from the endless realms of beings, one must focus attention with steadfastness: in that instant, whether in sleep or in the waking state, floods of merit, equal to the sky, begin to flow without ceasing. (verses 18–19)

The urge to liberation is a sign that a person's level of awareness has reached critical mass. He or she is no longer able to become unconscious, spiritually dull, but from now on there is a constant nagging sense of having to consciously cooperate in the evolutionary work.

In the Vedanta tradition, the urge to liberation is known as
mumukshutva, the desire for release from the fetters of karma. It is
considered to be a fundamental prerequisite on the spiritual path.
Without it, all one's ascetical practices remain barren.

The awakening of this urge can be seen as a kind of grace. It
places us into a completely different relationship to the world than
before. It opens our inner eyes. We become spiritual embryos.
Then during actual initiation, the second threshold, we are born as
spiritual beings. The subsequent progress is practically autonomous. The initiate or "stream entrant," to use the Buddhist expression, proceeds gradually along the various stages of maturation,
until there is full awakening.

But this awakening is preceded by our symbolic death
through consistent and demanding self-transcending practice,
which breaks down the self-will. Yet, far from leading to psychotic
collapse, this systematic deconstruction of the personality frees
our energy and attention for the realization of the ultimate Reality.
With the onset of enlightenment, the process triggered by the initial crisis fulfills itself. The circle is complete.

NOTES

1. On the psychology of Arjuna see the excellent study by G.W.
Kaveeshwar, *The Ethics of the Gita* (Delhi: Motilal Banarsidass, 1971), pp.
1–145.

2. S. Radhakrishnan, *The Bhagavadgita* (London: Allen & Unwin, 1948), p.
51.

3. *The Rig-Veda* (X.135) refers to the story of a boy who visits the realm of
Yama, Lord of Death. The fourteenth-century commentator Sayana identified the boy as Naciketas.

4. This is a summary paraphrase of several chapters, in which Prince
Rama explains himself.

CHAPTER 10

INITIATION AS SPIRITUAL REBIRTH

THE TRIAL OF INITIATION

All spiritual teachings are esoteric in nature. They are transmitted from an adept to a qualified disciple by way of mouth. At first, however, the teacher ascertains very carefully the spiritual aptitude of the aspirants. When they show the necessary qualities of determination, courage, and endurance, as well as physical and mental fitness, the teacher declares his or her readiness to instruct them, either formally or by silent consent.

The pact between teacher and disciple is consolidated during actual initiation, called *diksha* or *samskara* in Sanskrit. In some cases, novices must first undergo a certain period of probation, which is designed more to strengthen their intention and willpower than to supply the teacher with further proof of their qualification. The *Kula-Arnava-Tantra* (XIV.19), for instance, contains the following stipulation:

> A teacher should test the disciple in knowledge and in deed for a full year, or half of that [period], or [at least] half of that.

Longer trial periods were not uncommon. This point is made in a legend that is told in the ancient *Chandogya-Upanishad* (VIII.7ff.). Here God Indra and the Anti-God Virocana went to the Creator, Prajapati, for instruction. They were obliged to live with Prajapati for thirty-two years before he asked them what they desired in their life. Testing them, Prajapati gave them a false teaching. While Virocana proudly returned to his host of Anti-Gods with his new-found wisdom, Indra was not so taken in.

"Fuel in hand," he beseeched Prajapati to instruct him further. The Lord of Creation demanded that Indra live with him another thirty-two years. Again, Prajapati communicated to his disciple only half the truths at the end of the period. After thinking over the new teaching, Indra was again dissatisfied, requesting to be taught more. He had to wait another thirty-two years before the next instruction, which again turned out to be less than the truth. Finally, after having spent a total of 101 years in Prajapati's company and service, Indra was initiated into the secret teaching of the single Reality. The Lord of Creation addressed his worthy disciple thus:

> O Bounteous one, verily, this body is mortal. It is subject to death. Yet, it serves as the basis for that deathless, bodiless Self. Verily, the embodied one is subject to desirable and undesirable [experiences]. Verily, for the embodied one there is no freedom from desirable and undesirable [experiences]. [But] the Bodiless one, verily, is not in contact with desirable or undesirable [conditions]. (VIII.12.1)

The bodiless Self transcends both pleasure and pain, because it transcends all the possible conditions that give rise to those experiences. This esoteric doctrine forms the foundation of Vedanta metaphysics. Indra, and thousands of other spiritual aspirants, had to earn the privilege of hearing this liberating teaching.

Who does not remember the moving story of the Tibetan adept Milarepa? During his many years of discipleship under Marpa the Translator, who was a hard taskmaster, Milarepa was exposed to no end of trials and tribulations. Despite Milarepa's exemplary behavior, Marpa continued to refuse him initiation. It was only after Milarepa had been plunged into utter despair that his teacher finally, and still seemingly grudgingly, agreed to initiate him. It was all a test, of course. Later, Marpa reassured Milarepa that his, Marpa's, constant anger toward him had been an act.

Marpa's own pupilage under Naropa had been no less challenging, and Naropa's trials under Tilopa are legendary. While these stories are for the most part only stories, they capture the spirit of traditional discipleship very well. It was always an all-or-nothing affair. Disciples had to be prepared if necessary to die for the wisdom they were seeking. They understood that instruction and initiation were forms of spiritual empowerment, which would firmly place them on the path to freedom. The verbal teachings were not just intellectually stimulating considerations, and the initiatory ceremonies were not just intriguing rituals. They carried with them the force of truth.

Under certain circumstances, a teacher may consider an aspirant fit for instant initiation and empowerment. One of the best known examples is that of Swami Vivekananda. He was initiated on his second visit to the saintly Sri Ramakrishna, when he was still very much in doubt about this great teacher. At the time, Ramakrishna was alone, sitting on his bed. He invited Vivekananda to sit near him. Then he quickly touched him with his right foot.

At the touch, Vivekananda was hurled into a strange mystical state in which the whole universe and himself vanished into an all-engulfing Void. Fearfully he cried out: "What are you doing to me? I have my parents at home." Ramakrishna only laughed, touched Vivekananda's chest, and said: "All right, let us leave it there for the present. Everything will come in time." Instantly, Vivekananda returned to his ordinary consciousness. But he had been deeply affected, and he was drawn back to the saint.

On his third visit, Vivekananda tried his best to avoid physical contact with Ramakrishna; but before he knew it, the saint had touched him again, and this time he was plunged into a state in which there was no outward awareness left. Later Ramakrishna explained that he had put certain questions to Vivekananda while he was thus abstracted from the world. The young man's answers had confirmed the saint's intuitive knowledge about Vivekananda's spiritual past. Apparently he had been a realized master in his previous incarnation. Ramakrishna would say no more about it, but prophesied that Vivekananda would drop his body as soon as he remembered his true nature.

Swami Vivekananda died in 1902 at the age of thirty-nine. One evening, after meditating for an hour, he lay down, having a disciple fan his head. An hour later, his hands trembled slightly and he heaved two heavy breaths, exiting the body in yogic fashion. He had fulfilled his own frequent prophecy that he would not live to see forty. Possibly, he also fulfilled the prophecy of his teacher.

Any genuine initiation is always a charismatic act, in which the adepts implant part of their spiritual power into the being of the novice so that his or her endeavors may bear fruit. Symbolically, initiation is a birth act. As is stated in the ancient *Atharva-Veda* (XI.5.3):

> Initiation takes place in that the teacher carries the pupil in himself as it were, as the mother [bears] the embryo in her body. After the three days of the ceremony, the disciple is born.

Initiation effects a spiritual rebirth. Having renounced mundane life, the initiate now awakens to a new, higher reality. The initiatory rebirth is the germinal point of a long and comprehensive course of conversion, which reaches its peak when the now accomplished adept has fully transcended the world of phenomena. Through initiation, the aspirant becomes a member of a powerful chain of tradition, which may extend over many generations of teachers. From then on, teaching and teacher are to the spiritual practitioner as father and mother. As the Buddhist *Hevajra-Tantra* (II.4.61–62) states:

> The school is said to be the body. The monastery is called the womb. Through freedom from attachment, one is in the womb. The yellow robe is the membrane [around the embryo]. And the preceptor is [one's] mother. The salutation is the head-first position. Discipleship is [one's] worldly experience. And recitation of *mantras* is the [sense of] "I."

THE TEACHER AS THE GATEWAY TO REALITY

In exchange for the wisdom and experience received through the teaching and the teacher, the novice is expected to show great respect toward both and to do his or her utmost to prove worthy of initiation, instruction, and empowerment. To receive spiritual gnosis at the hands of an adept is a rare privilege and opportunity. As the *Shiva-Samhita* (III.1), a late manual on Hatha-Yoga, declares:

> Only the knowledge that comes from the mouth of the teacher is alive. Other kinds [of knowledge] are barren, powerless, and the cause of suffering.

The consensus in the spiritual traditions is that without a teacher, salvation is unattainable. In the *Mundaka-Upanishad* (I.2), we read:

For the realization of this [Self], [a seeker] should approach, fuel in hand, a teacher who is well-versed [in the scriptures] and established in the Absolute. To such a one who duly approaches [the teacher] and is tranquil-minded and peaceful, [the adept] imparts truthfully the knowledge of the Absolute so that he may realize the imperishable, true Self.

The ancient Hindu custom of bringing fuel-sticks to the teacher is a symbolic act by which aspirants offer their own body-minds as kindling for the great spiritual fire that only the adept can light in them. Only the teacher knows the path to the Light, for he has himself walked it successfully. The *Rig-Veda* (X.32.7) contains this verse:

One who does not know a country, asks one who knows it. Then, after having been informed by a knowledgeable [person], he travels [safely toward his destination].

As the Sanskrit word *guru* suggests, the teacher is "weighty." His or her experience and judgement are instrumental to the disciple's spiritual success. According to an esoteric etymology found in the *Saura-Purana* (LXVIII.10), the term guru signifies the following:

The sound *gu* is dark; the sound *ru* obstructing; the word *guru* hence is thus called because it obstructs darkness.

The same scripture (LXVIII.11), which has a strong sectarian orientation, contains this stern warning:

May he who deserts his teacher meet his death; may he who discontinues [the recitation of] the *mantras* become poverty-stricken; may he who deserts both, even if he were perfected, be cast into hell.

Traditionally, the *guru* is guardian, confidant, teacher, and judge in one person. In later times, the disciple was even asked to

regard the teacher as a divinity and serve him or her with unconditional devotion (*bhakti*). The guru acts as a constant monitor of the
supreme ideal of the renunciation of the ego. The guru is the great
archetype, which is to be imitated in one's discipleship.

The practice of *guru-yoga* consists in the worship of the Divine
in and through the person of the teacher. This has often led to all
sorts of excesses, both on the part of power-hungry teachers and
on the part of their immature disciples. However, even at the best
of times, guru-yoga has proven to be a rather risky path, as disciples are asked to focus exclusively on one person. Since disciples
are, by definition, spiritual children and dependent on the guru's
grace, they are apt to project onto him all their childish hopes and
fears. The guru then is worshipped as the ultimate savior, which is
precisely the central credo of guru-yoga.

The spiritual osmosis between teacher and disciple can happen only when the latter completely surrenders to the guru. It
takes a very wise and compassionate teacher not to get entrapped
in this process, and a very mature disciple not to delude himself or
herself.

Contemporary attempts to revive this archaic form of spiritual
practice by adepts teaching in the West must be seen as false starts.
They inevitably lead to a counterproductive personality cult in
which the guru is turned into a golden calf, while the disciples exchange an attitude of generic obedience for personal responsibility.
The danger of such an approach has been amply demonstrated by
the Rajneeshie cult, which gave rise to militant sectarianism.

Our Western personality, rooted as it is in the mental structure
of consciousness, is ill-suited for monolithic surrender of the type
called for in traditional guru-yoga. The kind of exclusive devotion
called for in guru-yoga manifests the longing of the mythic consciousness for self-effacement and self-denial. In more integral
spiritual approaches, we can expect the relationship between
teacher and disciple to be far more open, dialectical, and non-
exclusive.

CHAPTER 11

THE PATH FROM MULTIPLICITY TO UNITY

THE EIGHT LIMBS OF YOGIC UNIFICATION

So far we have examined the most essential features of mythic spirituality—its bipolar approach, escape from time, denigration of ego-self and world, perception of suffering in everything, and cyclic outlook on life. The following chapters will discuss in more concrete detail the actual path of spiritual unification. The focus of attention will be on the eightfold path of Classical Yoga, as developed by Patanjali in the *Yoga-Sutra*.

This scripture, which consists of 195 aphorisms (*sutra*), was probably composed some time around 200 A.D. It provides a reasonably systematic treatment of the philosophical tenets and fundamental practices of Patanjali's school. However, the style in which it is written is so terse that it is at times difficult to know exactly what the author had in mind. Luckily, we have several ancient Sanskrit commentaries that shed some light on these obscurities.

It is evident from the *Yoga-Sutra* that Patanjali did not originate Yoga philosophy. He merely tried to systematize it, and there are a number of aphorisms that appear to be quoted from another scripture which is no longer extant. Patanjali arranged the yogic path into eight "limbs" (*anga*).

An older model is the "six-member Yoga" (*shad-anga-yoga*) laid down in the *Maitrayaniya-Upanishad*, a work belonging to the pre-Christian era. It is remarkable insofar as it does not itemize the first three limbs of Classical Yoga as separate components, namely ethical discipline (*yama*), self-restraint (*niyama*), and posture (*asana*). Instead, it has a new element called *tarka*, which was probably inspired by Buddhism. This appears to be the practice of critically inspecting the higher mystical experiences.

Other variants of the yogic path, with ten, fifteen, or more limbs, are also known. However, these are not important to the present consideration.

Patanjali's popular eight-limbed model comprises the following members:

1. *yama* — "restraint," in the sense of general ethical discipline
2. *niyama* — self-discipline
3. *asana* — posture
4. *pranayama* — regulation of breath/life energy (*prana*)
5. *pratyahara* — withdrawal of the senses
6. *dharana* — concentration
7. *dhyana*— meditative absorption
8. *samadhi* — ecstatic unification

These are the constituent practices of Classical Yoga. The vertical arrangement, however, is only conditionally justified. It would be misleading to interpret these practices as stages, as is commonly done. Rather, they should be compared with functional units that overlap both chronologically and operationally. So, for instance, the first two limbs are clearly practiced together, and sensory inhibition, concentration, and meditation must also be regarded as pertaining to one and the same process of introversion. Hence a circular arrangement suggests itself.

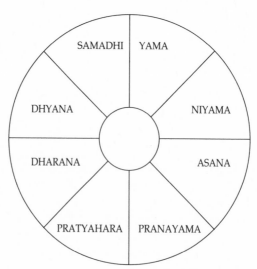

The above diagrammatic representation shows very clearly the existing relationship between the various members. Thus, yama has pratyahara as its opposite, which bears out its exact function on the social level, for yama in the last analysis is the abstention from encroaching on the life-space of others. Niyama aptly faces dharana, since it is essentially ethical "concentration." Asana lies opposite dhyana, which reminds us that posture is basically a meditative attitude of the body. Pranayama, again, has samadhi as its counterpart, which hints at the mediating function of both: While the former mediates on the physical level between internal and external reality by means of the activity of the life energy, the latter acts as mediator between the phenomenal and the transcendental Reality.

The dynamic tension between the eight limbs creates "upward" acceleration and is responsible for the ultimate exit from conditioned existence. Accordingly, the center of the circle is assigned to the goal of Yoga.

The creative tension inherent in the spiritual process is emphasized by the author of the *Yoga-Kundalini-Upanishad* (III.14b–15) as follows:

> As the flame, dormant in the wood, cannot flare up without friction, so also the torch of gnosis [cannot shine] without Yoga practice.

The yogin's intense concern for unification manifests itself unmistakeably in all the techniques and on all levels of the yogic enterprise. Every exercise and effort is aimed at centering the psyche and all its outgoing activities. In his erudite study on Yoga, Mircea Eliade rightly observed that "the tendency toward 'unification' and 'totalization' is a feature of all yogic techniques."[1]

The first task of this extensive process of reversal and introversion is the harmonization of one's relationships with the environment. The necessary momentum for this obligation is provided by one's imitation of the transcendental Reality, which knows no distinctions. This *imitatio Dei*, or duplication of the suprahuman, supramundane Being can be met everywhere in Yoga. The following words of the divine teacher Krishna exemplify this approach:

But those who worship the imperishable, indefinable Unmanifest, which is omnipresent, unthinkable, summit-abiding
(*kuta-stha*), unmoving, and firm . . . they attain to Me.[2]

Here the yogins are urged to orientate their every thought and
wish toward the One that surpasses all opposites, and to repro-
duce it, as it were, in miniature within themselves. The ascetics
project themselves, at first purely intellectually, into the un-
fractured transcendental Oneness and from there draw the energy
and strength necessary to effect the desired unification of their
psyche. Thus they are capable of restraining their greed for life, of
freeing themselves from the coercion of the instincts, and of adopting a benevolent attitude toward all beings. Of course, in mythic
Yoga the emphasis is not so much on active charity as on the avoid-
ance of doing harm to others, which is a more passive virtue.

SPIRITUAL DISCIPLINE AS REVERSAL

From what has been said so far it is evident that any genuine
yogic act always goes against the grain of conventional life. It represents a deliberate opposition to unenlightened existence. The
yogins do on all levels of human existence the opposite of what life
demands. As Mircea Eliade noted, "The 'reversal' of normal
behaviour sets the yogin outside life. But he does not stop half-
way—death is followed by an initiatory re-birth."[3]

This yogic reversal of ordinary behavior is most strikingly apparent, on the physical level, in the bodily posture called *viparita-
karani*, or "inverted practice," that is, the headstand.[4] Not surprisingly, this posture has become the symbol for Yoga in the popular
understanding of the West.

The yogin's opposition must not be construed to mean a mor-
bid hatred of life. Any such emotion would be detrimental to the
spiritual process. Rather, it is a positive force, which has its roots in
a vision that penetrates through the surface reality of life. The yogic aspirants seek to model their life after the great archetype of the
One beyond the Many. Their opposition to conditioned existence is
the inevitable result of their endeavor to actualize the Unconditioned.

The representatives of the mythic orientation within the Yoga movement have typically pursued this goal with a precarious onesidedness. Their rejection of ordinary life has often been so radical as to be questionable. In some cases, the denial of the body, for instance, has been pushed to such extremes that their practice resembled fakirism rather than Yoga. At times, we must even suspect the presence of a strong neurosis. Only the most mature individuals are able to safely negotiate the pitfalls of radical approaches to spirituality.

All spiritual work entails the risk of being thrown off balance. Therefore the authoritative texts without exception emphasize that only the most vital, intelligent, and courageous practitioners are likely to succeed. Thus, the *Mahabharata* epic (XII.300,50) contains this verse:

> This great path of the wise brahmins is difficult [to follow]. No one can tread it easily, O Bharatarishabha! It resembles a terrifying jungle creeping with great serpents, [filled] with [innumerable] pits, devoid of water, full of thorns and inaccessible [to all but the strongest].

NOTES

1. M. Eliade, Yoga: *Immortality and Freedom* (Princeton, NJ: Princeton University Press, 1970), p. 55.

2. *Bhagavad-Gita* XII.4.

3. M. Eliade, *op. cit.*, p. 362.

4. For a clarification of the nature of this exercise, see G. Feuerstein "The Inverted Pose (*Viparita-Karani-Mudra*) According to the Sanskrit Texts," *The Yoga Review: Quarterly Journal of the Indian Academy of Yoga*, vol. 2, no. 2 (1982), pp. 79–87.

CHAPTER 12

THE PURITAN ETHICS

THE REGULATION OF SOCIAL ACTION

The first two members of the spiritual path, as taught by Patanjali, are moral discipline (yama) and self-restraint (niyama). Some scholars have claimed these to be later additions. However, this claim rests on a profound misunderstanding of the structure of the yogic path. Even where these two "limbs" are not listed separately, they nevertheless are an integral part of the spiritual aspirant's endeavor.

The Czech scholar Adolf Janáček was the first to refute this mistaken scholarly assumption. He demonstrated that these two categories of Yoga share the same underlying principle that can also be shown in the case of the other limbs: the principle of cultivating the opposite, or *pratipaksha-bhavana*.[1]

This Sanskrit expression appears in the *Yoga-Sutra* (II.33) in connection with the treatment of the faulty attitudes (*vitarka*), such as the intentions "I shall kill him who hurt me," "I shall appropriate his possessions, too," "I shall also tell a lie," etc.[2] These perverse thoughts end in the experience of suffering and in still deeper spiritual delusion. It does not even matter whether they have been executed or have incited others to action, or even whether they have merely been tolerated.

The spiritual practitioner must at all events prevent any thoughts or intentions that are antagonistic to the spiritual work. Patanjali's recommended procedure for blocking out dissonant thoughts is the absorption of the mind into their exact opposites, that is, the kindling and cultivation of thoughts of peacefulness and truth.

The first member of the eightfold path, yama, regulates the aspirant's external activity. The word comes from the verbal root *yam* ("to hold up, sustain") and can appropriately be rendered as "restraint" or "discipline." Often the term is also translated as "moral observance."

The *Yoga-Sutra* (II.30) mentions and defines the following five constituent practices of yama.

1. *ahimsa* — nonharming
2. *satya* — truthfulness
3. *asteya* — nonstealing
4. *brahmacarya* — chastity
5. *aparigraha* — greedlessness

According to Patanjali's aphorism II.31, these constitute the "great vow" (*maha-vrata*) and must be practiced regardless of place, time, circumstances, and one's particular position in life. In other words, they have universal validity. They are meant to uproot mainly the two most powerful human urges, that of sexuality and that of domination. Should this fundamental step not be taken, the insubordinate instinctual life would cause growing psychomental confusion and disintegration.

In particular, the magical powers acquired in the higher stages of the spiritual path would be in danger of being subordinated to the fulfillment of one's lower instincts. This would lead to their gross abuse, to the detriment of others as well as oneself. On the other hand, conscientious observation of these ethical rules bestows on the aspirant the essential moral stability without which he or she would be at the mercy of the dangers of a licentious sorcerdom. Again and again, the Yoga texts emphasize that moral integrity is an indispensable precondition of spiritual success. The acquisition of power must be counterbalanced by a simultaneous growth of one's sense of responsibility.

True as it is that the mythic yogins endeavor to withdraw from social life, seeking their good in almost hermetic seclusion, they are nonetheless concerned with making their relationships to other beings as harmonious as possible. However, this is not primarily for any ethical reasons, but simply in recognition of the fact that there is only the One and that any feeling or thought of otherness or antagonism would blatantly contradict this great truth and prove detrimental to the work of unification. Only by seeking the One in the Many can it be found beyond the Many.

The five rules comprised by moral discipline are basic ethical requirements and in one form or another are present in all higher religions. To the Hindu they are reflections of the cosmic order (dharma or rita) without which we could never attain liberation. As Mircea Eliade remarked:

> The "restraints" produce not a yogic state but a "purified" human being, superior to the ordinary run. This purity is essential to the succeeding stages.[3]

NONHARMING AND THE OTHER VIRTUES

The most important ethical precept, which supports all others, is that of nonharming or *ahimsa*. As the South Indian saint Tiru-Valluvar affirms in his *Tiru-Kural* (321), a work consisting of 1330 stanzas and reverentially called the "Tamil Veda":

> The greatest virtue is nonharming; [deliberate] harming [of other beings] brings in its wake all other evils.

In his *Yoga-Bhashya* (II.30), the oldest extant commentary on the Yoga aphorisms, Vyasa elucidates:

> Nonharming is the unconditional nonhurting (*anabhi-droha*) of any being at all times. And in this are rooted the other disciplines and restraints, and they serve the perfection of this [precept], and its illustration.

From this it is clear that nonharming entails much more than is borne out by the usual rendering of this Sanskrit term as "nonkilling." It means nonviolence in the widest possible sense—in thoughts and in deeds. It is, as the *Mahabharata* (III.312.76) confirms, nonmaliciousness (*anrishamsya*) in the sense of abiding kindness.

This virtue is the best illustration of the fact that the chosen encapsulation of yogins must not be viewed as a mere *egotistic* escape from mundane concerns; their unitive life has a purifying effect on the environment. For, as the *Yoga-Sutra* (II.35) states, in the proximity of a person grounded in this virtue no feeling of enmity can arise. The lucid, peaceful aura of adepts averts all strife, and even the most ferocious animals lose their instinct to kill when near such saintly folk. In addition, if we can believe the physician Caraka, one of the great lights of India's native medicine, hurting others reduces one's lifespan, whereas nonharming helps to prolong it.

The virtue of nonharming reached its most exalted position in Jainism, whose founder, Mahavira, is said to have placed his feet on the ground only after he had made quite sure that no animal would be killed. The canonical texts also relate that his body housed whole colonies of insects, which he refused to destroy or even remove lest they should be harmed. Even today the Jaina monks and nuns eat only in broad daylight to prevent unintentionally swallowing an insect. It is self-evident that vegetarianism is the only authorized form of nourishment.

The contrast between the Jaina monk's attitude of nonharming, or internalized sacrifice, and the sacrificial ritualism of the Hindu brahmins is strikingly highlighted in the following story.

One day, the Jaina monk Harikesha, who had just completed a long fast, went begging for alms among the brahmins. Before his conversion to Jainism, he had been a member of the lowest caste of Hindu society. Since he was an ascetic of some renown, his previous history was also well known to the local people. So, when he entered the precincts of a group of brahmins who had gathered to perform an animal sacrifice, he was welcomed with abuse.

When Harikesha reminded the brahmins that their behavior was unbecoming of saintly folk, they rushed forward and beat him with sticks. They were prevented from doing the sage serious harm only because a demi-god appeared and warned them off. Seeing the apparition who had come to Harikesha's defense, the brahmins became quite contrite. The sage generously forgave them and then proceeded to instruct them in the art of true sacrifice. He taught them that slaughtering animals or even taking ritual baths in the river have nothing to do with sacrifice. True sacrifice, he explained, consists in preserving one's purity by strictly observing the moral rules that prevent the creation of karma.

The virtue of truthfulness (*satya*) is likewise connected with the acquisition of a special power: Whatever the practitioner established in this virtue pronounces will inevitably come true.[4] From earliest times, truthfulness has been praised as a great source of strength. It is truth that is said to sustain the universe. This ancient conviction is emphasized by the author of the *Mahanirvana-Tantra* (IV.75–77) in the following passage:

> No virtue is more excellent than truthfulness, no sin greater than [telling] the untruth. Therefore the [virtuous] man should seek refuge in truthfulness with all his heart. Without truthfulness, worship is futile; without truthfulness, the recitation [of sacred mantras] is useless; without truthfulness, austerities are as unfruitful as seed on barren land. Truthfulness is the form of the supreme Absolute. Truthfulness truly is the best asceticism. All deeds [should be] rooted in truthfulness, nothing is more excellent than truthfulness.

The virtue of nonstealing (*asteya*), the third of the precepts included in yama, is intimately linked with the demand for desisting from hankering after another's property, or *aparigraha*. When the aspirant has fully acquired the virtue of nonstealing, all kinds of treasures are said to accrue to him or her effortlessly.[5] The virtue of greedlessness, again, leads to knowledge about one's former existences.[6]

Finally, the virtue of chastity, to which special importance is attached, remains to be considered. The term *brahmacarya* literally means "moving in the Absolute" or "brahmanic conduct." This is suggestive of the fundamental practice of imitating the transcendental Reality in one's actions. Thus, the aspirants endeavor to actualize the mode of the One in all their activities. That is to say, they attempt to live continually in the light of the Absolute. The *Darshana-Upanishad* (I.13–14), a relatively recent work that interprets Yoga from the perspective of Vedanta nondualism, contains the following explanation of *brahmacarya*:

> Perfect abstention from women in body, speech and mind, with the exception of one's own wife in the prescribed manner—that is called "chastity." The orientation of the mind toward the state of the Absolute is *brahmacarya*, O Paramtapa!

Thus, the anonymous author of the *Darshana-Upanishad* interprets chastity more as an inner attitude than as a fixed set of practices. Writing for the householder who is engaged in spiritual life, he allows sex with one's own wife, but only in accordance with the established norms. This excludes sexual intercourse during menstruation—an important taboo for pious Hindus as well as many other traditional cultures.

The strict ascetic view is put forward in the *Shandilya-Upanishad* (I.I.8), another medieval work:

Abstention from intercourse in thoughts, words and deeds, everywhere and under any circumstances is what is called "chastity."

The yogins who practice chastity gain great bodily and mental vitality, which enables them to restrain the senses and to rush toward the goal of the Self with concentrated mind, whereas sexuality is a gate to death. In a similar vein, the *Yoga-Sutra* (II.38) states:

[One's being] grounded in chastity [leads to] the attainment of vitality.

Vyasa comments on this:

Through the attainment of this [vitality], one increases one's unobstructed [magical] abilities, and [if one is] an adept, one becomes competent to transfer one's knowledge to disciples.[7]

The *Prashna-Upanishad* (V.5), a pre-Christian scripture, declares:

As a serpent casts off its old skin, so the yogin frees himself from all sin through the diligent observation of chastity.

We encounter the expression "brahmacarya" as far back as the early *Upanishads*, where it signifies the years of apprenticeship in the life of the orthodox Hindu. In the course of time, it obtained the specific meaning of "chastity," which evinces the great importance attached to this cardinal virtue. The idea of chastity as a spiritual discipline is, however, much older still. This is exemplified by a remarkable hymn of the *Rig-Veda* (I.179), which records an

intimate conversation between the ascetic Agastya and his wife
Lopamudra.

Having become weary of sexual abstinence, Lopamudra sets
out to seduce her husband who, after some initial qualms, capitu-
lates and yields to his lust. Feeling great compunction, Agastya re-
sorts to the purifying *soma* sacrifice to restore his inner balance. We
can readily imagine that this story had its historical basis in the
experience of more than a few Vedic households.

THE FATEFUL CONSEQUENCES OF IMMORALITY

The five moral precepts are designed to purify the mind and
effectively block the three "gates to hell," namely sensual desire,
anger, and greed. They represent the first step toward the transformation of the individual by putting an end to heedlessness and
neurotic compulsive acts. The character and fate of those who fail
to observe these basic moral virtues, which constitute the mini-
mum of any humanistic ethics, is vividly described in the
Bhagavad-Gita (XVI.6ff.):

> Two [types of] beings are in this world—the divine and the
> demoniac. The divine [I have already] explained extensively.
> Hear from Me [now] about the demoniac [beings], O son of
> Pritha. (6)

> The demoniac people do not know [the difference between
> worldly] activity and cessation. Neither purity nor good con-
> duct, nor truthfulness is found in them. (7)

> They say: "The world is devoid of truth, without foundation,
> without a lord, not produced in sequence; what else is it but
> desire-caused?" (8)

> Holding this view, these lost souls of little wisdom and
> cruel deeds, come forth as enemies for the destruction of the
> world. (9)

> Abandoning themselves to insatiable desire, possessed of os-
> tentation, pride and intoxication, holding untrue conceptions
> through delusion, they engage in impure vows. (10)

Obsessed with innumerable cares ending [only] with dissolution [at death], having the gratification of desires as their supreme [goal]—they are convinced that this [is all there is to life]. (11)

Bound by hundreds of cords of hope, addicted to desire and anger, they strive to amass wealth by unjust means, with the [sole] purpose of gratifying their desires. (12)

These cruel haters, vilest of men, and evil, I hurl [birth after birth] untiringly back into the cycle [of birth and death], into demoniac wombs. (19)

Fallen into demoniac wombs, birth after birth deluded, not reaching Me—[these unfortunate people] thence go to the lowest state, O son of Kunti. (20)

The "lowest state" is the hell realm. We can understand this as the condition of spiritual darkness, where individuals are trapped in their own subjective distortion of reality, far removed from the divine Light.

By observing the moral virtues recommended in all the great spiritual traditions of the world, this fall can be prevented. More than that, a virtuous life can serve as firm ground for realizing our higher evolutionary possibilities.

NOTES

1. See A. Janáček, "The Methodological Principle in Yoga," *Archiv Orientální*, vol. 19 (Prague, 1951), pp. 514–567.

2. See *Yoga-Bhashya* II.33.

3. M. Eliade, *Patanjali and Yoga* (New York: Schocken Books, 1975), p. 63.

4. See *Yoga-Sutra* II.36.

5. See *Yoga-Sutra* II.37.

6. See *Yoga-Sutra* II.39.

7. *Yoga-Bhashya* II.38.

CHAPTER 13

THE DENIAL OF EROS

SEX IS KARMIC

In the preceding chapter, we briefly looked at the virtue of chastity as an integral aspect of the spiritual path. This element deserves more careful consideration, as it is one of the most ideologically charged practices of mythic spirituality. The mythic orientation to life has a problem with embodiment, which is deemed unworthy and opposed to the Spirit. On the most elementary level, embodiment means sexuality. For it is through the sexual process that embodied beings perpetuate the species to which they belong.

In the case of human beings, the biological act of procreation is overlaid with all kinds of social and personal significances. Most notable is the idea that procreation not only ensures the survival of the race but offers the ordinary person a substitute for immortality: Men and women seek to perpetuate themselves in their children. For the world-denying mythic consciousness, this is a particularly potent and dangerous ideal. The danger lies in that it entices people to invest their attention and energy in finite pursuits rather than in the quest for the Infinite.

From the mythic viewpoint, sex is karmic. First, it acts as a powerful attractor between people, thus involving them in joint experiences that are seldom spiritually motivated. Second, it creates long-term material and social obligations that tend to divert people's attention from the spiritual realm. Hence the mythic consciousness is wary of marriage and romantic entanglements.

It is especially wary of the sex act itself because it entails a loss of psychosomatic energy. Orgasm is seen as the ultimate betrayal of spiritual principles. In orgasm, the ego-personality indulges in self-pleasuring, which has nothing to do with the ultimate bliss. It trades that eternal happiness for a few seconds of pleasurable thrill. In the process, it depletes its store of psychoenergy, thus diminishing its spiritual possibilities. For the spiritual process requires great vitality.

According to the *Shiva-Samhita* (V.75–76), a late work on Hatha-Yoga, the food we consume is broken down by our body into three forms. The best distillate goes to nourish our psychic field. The second-best extract feeds the body's seven physical constituents (bones, lymph, blood, marrow, tissue, fat, and semen). The third form is eliminated as feces and urine.

Orgasm, which is not only a discharge of semen but primarily a neurological event, throws off a great amount of energy from our psychic field. It is therefore thought to destabilize the psyche and to steal valuable nutrients from the physical body.

Spiritual aspirants within the mythic orientation are genuinely afraid of the loss of psychosomatic vitality. This fear is particularly strong in men, where orgasm involves the ejaculation of semen. Although women, too, secrete before and during orgasm, much of their vaginal fluid is reabsorbed by the body. Hence women were traditionally considered to have a distinct advantage over men.

The male concern is expressed, for instance, in the *Hatha-Yoga-Pradipika* (III.88). After describing a curious technique for sucking the semen back into the penis after ejaculation, Svatmarama, the author of this medieval work, states:

Thus, the knower of Yoga should preserve the semen (*bindu*). [Then] he conquers death. By ejaculating the semen, there is death. By preserving the semen, there is life.

The adept Svatmarama adds:

By preserving the semen, a pleasant smell is produced in the yogin's body. So long as the semen remains in the body, how can there be fear of death?

God Shiva declares in the *Shiva-Samhita* (IV.89–92):

There is no doubt that the world is born and dies by means of the semen. Knowing this, the yogin should always practice preservation of the semen.

When the semen has been controlled with great effort, how can one not control the world? By the grace of such [control], I myself have become like this!

The semen creates pleasure and pain for all those deluded worldlings who are subject to ageing and death.

[But] this is a beneficial Yoga for the most excellent yogins. Through practice, even the [ordinary] person hooked on [worldly] experiences attains control [over the semen].

God Shiva, who uttered these words, is the arch adept of mythical spirituality. He is the ascetic *par excellence*. Here he presents himself as a master of seminal control, attributing his elevated state to this esoteric practice.

Interestingly, this whole attitude has a striking parallel in Chinese Taoism. Here male adepts are instructed to retain the semen at all costs and, indeed, to have intercourse with healthy maidens so that they can even tap into the female vitality. Not without some justification, this practice has been labelled "spiritual vampirism." A similar practice is recommended in certain schools of Tantrism, which will be discussed in a later chapter.

WOMEN AS OBSTACLES ON THE SPIRITUAL PATH

Most traditional schools of spirituality evince a strong male bias. Seldom do their scriptures even take women into account, never mind featuring spiritual heroines. Indeed, for the patriarchal representatives of the mythic consciousness, women are dangerous. Gautama the Buddha is said to have admitted women only most reluctantly into his order. He reputedly even said that their admission would halve the lifespan of the Buddhist order.[1]

In Hindu society, at least in the North, women have traditionally been relegated to a status inferior to that of men. This attitude is epitomized in the juridical literature. Thus in the *Manu-Smriti* (V.147ff.), it is clearly spelled out that a woman is dependent first on her father and later on her husband and, upon the death of her spouse, on her children. This scripture also stipulates that a woman should always worship her husband as God, regardless of any shortcomings he may have.

In the religious literature, women are widely regarded as little more than sexual triggers. Thus, many texts contain shocking vituperations of the female gender. For instance, the author of the *Yoga-Vasishtha* (I.21.1ff.) put the following unflattering words into Prince Rama's mouth:

> What is so beautiful about a woman, who is but a fleshy doll in a cage of moving machinery composed of bones, joints, and sinews? (1)

> A woman's loveliness lasts only briefly. O sage, I deem her to be nothing but a cause of delusion. (8)

> Verily, women are fuel for the fire of hell. They burn even from afar. [They appear] charming but are insipid, and [seem] lovely but are severe. (12)

> O sage, this earth with its various experiences and different pleasures is dependent for its continued existence on women. (22)

> He who has a wife has a desire for enjoyment. But how can there be enjoyment for one who has no wife? To abandon a woman is to abandon the world. Upon abandoning the world, one becomes happy. (35)

It is not surprising that in the strongly patriarchal society of India the yogic scriptures should extol the advantages of a male embodiment. According to some misogynous extremists, liberation was not even possible for a woman. Thus, even an advanced female practitioner would have to be reborn as a man before attaining full enlightenment.

This is the viewpoint advocated, for instance, by the Digambara ("Sky-Clad") sect of Jainism. The Digambaras believe that women lack the adamantine body instrumental to the attainment of liberation. Women are even excluded from joining this sect, because they cannot meet the fundamental requirement of public nudity. The highly austere Digambaras have no possessions at all. They beg for their food only once a day, and any offerings they receive must be placed in their upturned palms.

The Shvetambara sect, which is the second great division

within Jainism, favors a more moderate approach. They admit women into their order, and even insist that Malli, the nineteenth "ford-maker" (*tirthankara*) or enlightened teacher of Jainism, was a woman. According to tradition, Malli was King Mahabala in her previous incarnation. That king, together with seven close friends, renounced the world to become Jaina monks. They swore a solemn oath to endure an identical number of severe fasts.

Mahabala, who wanted to pursue the ascetic life with the utmost rigor, broke the agreement by finding ways to fast more frequently than his friends. Even though his behavior was otherwise exemplary and qualified him for enlightenment in his next birth, the fact that in his enthusiasm he cheated his companions bore karmic consequences. He was promptly born with a female body.

In her youth, Malli, the reincarnated king, was wooed by many men. In fact, like Helen of Troy, her beauty even occasioned a war. Deploring the suffering caused on her behalf and weary of the lustful overtures of her suitors, Malli renounced the world. There is one sculpture, now headless, which shows her sitting cross-legged in the nude.

Most Indian authorities adopted a more moderate position than that espoused by the Digambara radicals. While the majority still considered women to be at a disadvantage in spiritual life, they at least conceded that a truly outstanding female adept could reach the highest goal in this lifetime. Although the Sanskrit literature mentions comparatively few female adepts by name, those who are referred to are presented as being equal to their male counterparts.

NOTE

1. This is a widely accepted interpretation. However, in his book *The Three Jewels* (London: Rider, 1967), Bhikshu Sangharakshita argues that a careful analysis of the canonical text does not support this popular reading.

CHAPTER 14

SELF-DISCIPLINE AS ENERGY MANAGEMENT

FROM SIN TO PURE SELFHOOD

The second limb of Classical Yoga continues the process of "harnessing" the aspirant's psychic energy, which was initiated by the practice of the five basic moral virtues. The conservation of energy is a foremost obligation for the spiritual aspirant. As the contemporary Yoga master Swami Shivananda observed:

> Many do not know how to conserve the energy and regulate it according to the needs. They do not know how to transmute one form of energy into another form. That is why the vast majority of persons are not able to become prodigies or geniuses in the world. If you really want to become a great man, if you want to achieve something grand and sublime, conservation of energy will help you a lot. . . . A Yogi or a Jnani [sage] does not allow even a very small amount of energy in him to be wasted in useless directions.[1]

As we have seen, the quintuple rules of moral discipline (yama) are designed to regulate, or harmonize, the practitioner's energies in regard to his or her social interaction. This frees up energy for the more demanding spiritual practices of self-restraint (niyama). According to the *Yoga-Sutra* (II.32), the five restraints are as follows:

1. *shauca* — purity
2. *samtosha* — contentment
3. *tapas*— asceticism
4. *svadhyaya* — self-study
5. *ishvara-pranidhana* — devotion to the Lord

Later scriptures mention ten restraints. For instance, the *Hatha-Yoga-Pradipika* (I.16) lists asceticism, contentment, loyalty to the

orthodox tradition (*astikya*), charity, worship of God, listening to
the exposition of the doctrine, modesty, discernment, recitation of
mantras, and sacrifice. However, Patanjali's model commends itself for its simplicity.

The five component disciplines of this second limb of the yogic path have the purpose of accelerating the development of inwardness. The first two elements—purity and contentment—provide a transition from the level of external or social relationships to
the more advanced disciplines.

Thus, purity (shauca) creates a certain inner distance from
one's own body. This is the art of witnessing the body-mind without becoming constantly implicated in its functions. The Sanskrit
term employed for this detached attitude is *jugupsa*, which is usually rendered a "disgust" but more properly signifies something
much more positive. The word stems from the verbal root *gup*
meaning "to protect, guard" and hence is more correctly translated
as "being on one's guard" against the body-mind.

As has been explained already, the mythic consciousness experiences the body as an intruder, a disruptive force. For this reason,
representatives of this orientation always endeavor to neutralize
the influence of the body-mind.

The purification practices demonstrate to aspirants the basic
impurity of the body, and kindle in them a desire for that inner
purity that results from the purging of all spiritual blemishes. They
lose their attachment to the body and awaken to the dazzling possibilities of higher consciousness.

The purification practices hold before them the opportunity to
conquer their fateful identification with the physical body, which
is the greatest obstruction to the realization of the Self. The cultivation of inner and bodily purity heightens the sensitivity of practitioners to such a degree that they experience any contact with ordinary people as polluting. Hence they prefer to work in silent seclusion.

From the above it should be clear that shauca entails much
more than mere bodily cleanliness. As the sage Markandeya points
out in the *Mahabharata* epic (III.199.82), shauca means purity in
speech and deeds, as well as purification by physical means such
as water. This is the chastening of one's whole being in every

sense. According to the *Yoga-Sutra* (II.41), it leads to the purification of the personality core (*sattva*) itself. One of the aphorisms (III.55) indicates that when the personality core abides in the same pure condition as the Self, the adept achieves emancipation. In a way, the spiritual path is nothing but a systematic and comprehensive process of catharsis. Profane individuals are thought to live in a continual state of impurity and sin (papa). Their lowly condition is the outcome of their progressive secession from the transcendental Origin over many births. In fact, sin is just this separation from the ultimate Being. It is the state of self-contraction.

Yoga, like all other forms of mysticism, attempts to put a stop to this separative movement and to lead the human being back to the primordial Reality. All-out purification is the *modus operandi* by which recovery of the Origin is sought.

The *Manu-Smriti* (V.109), the most important and earliest metrical work on law, ethics, and conduct, specifies the various levels of purification as follows:

> The body is cleansed by water; the mind is purified by truthfulness; the personality essence (*bhuta-atman*) is purified by wisdom and austerities, and intelligence (*buddhi*) by [higher] knowledge.

On the higher level, purification thus involves liberating gnosis. The whole point of the spiritual program of catharsis is to recapture the original State of eternal purity. In essence we are already pure. To think otherwise is precisely the great fallacy of the unenlightened individual. As the *Darshana-Upanishad* (V.14) puts it:

> He alone who washes away the mire of nescience with the water of gnosis is ever pure, but not he who delights in [mundane] activity.

This sentiment is reiterated in Shankara's *Atma-Bodha* (66) as follows:

> Heated in the fire of gnosis and fanned by listening [to the sacred scriptures] and by the other [means to liberation], one's

psyche (*jiva*) shines forth in itself, devoid of any taints, like [pure] gold.

Just as the unpurified mind can never grasp the utter transparency and luminosity of the Self, so the mind unruffled by worldly concerns naturally reflects the tranquil light of the supreme Being-Awareness. In the succinct formulation of the author of the *Maitrayaniya-Upanishad* (VI.34), we learn

> . . . that the mind is said to be twofold: pure and impure. It is impure from contact with desires; pure when freed from desire. When one has liberated the mind from slothfulness and heedlessness and made it immovable and then attains to the mindless [state], this is the supreme estate. The mind should be restrained within until it becomes dissolved. This is gnosis and salvation; all else is but book knowledge. He whose mind has become pure through absorption and entered the Self, experiences a bliss impossible to describe in words and only intelligible to the inner instrument.

The "dissolution" of the mind mentioned in the above passage must not be understood as a psychotic breakdown. Rather, it refers to an important phase in the spiritual process in which the mind is transcended. Unenlightened individuals identify with "their" mind in the same way in which they identify with "their" body. In their day-to-day life, they rarely merely witness the activities of the body-mind. In other words, they seldom identify with the Spirit, or Self, which transcends all bodily and mental states.

As spiritual practitioners make progress on the path, they learn above all to disentangle themselves from their psychosomatic reactions. Increasingly, they position themselves in the transcendental witness, the Self. To express this more accurately, they *are* increasingly present as that Self.

To the extent that aspirants can free themselves from the deep-rooted notions of "I" and "mine," they secure for themselves the virtue of contentment (samtosha). This is a pervasive mood, which reflects the stillness of the transcendental Self.

Without contentment, or elated serenity, success on the spiritual path is unthinkable. A mind that harbors gloomy moods and is upset by doubts and misgivings is unfit for this great work. Only a positive, settled frame of mind is conducive to inner strength and the attainment of higher states of consciousness. As the *Mahabharata* (XII.21.2) puts it:

Contentment is indeed the highest heaven. Contentment is supreme joy. There is no higher satisfaction. It is complete in itself.

Ordinarily we react to our environment more or less mechanically, without much conscious participation. Our reactivity then sets in motion a whole chain reaction of undesirable mental states, which can be brought under control only with the greatest difficulty. Mature spiritual practitioners, by contrast, expect nothing from outside; they are self-sufficient, and therefore nothing can disappoint or upset them. Whatever they may encounter, their inner equilibrium remains stable.

Samtosha, or contentment, is closely linked with the important practice of equanimity (samatva), as recommended in the *Bhagavad-Gita* (II.48). Equanimity has several grades of intensity and levels of application. First of all, it is the quality of perfect indifference with regard to material things and values. Adepts are as indifferent to a piece of gold as they are to a lump of earth.

Equanimity also stands for that state of mind in which one remains unaffected by sorrow and pleasure, success and failure, praise and blame—in short, by the ups and downs of life. Finally, on the highest level, it is the all-embracing vision of sameness (*sama-darshana*), which reveals to adepts the ultimate Being wherever their glance may fall. In the words of the *Bhagavad-Gita* (VI.29):

He whose self is yoked in Yoga and who everywhere beholds the same, sees the Self abiding in all beings and all beings in the Self.

True practitioners are content with what accrues to them from life. The more they eradicate their self-will (*ahamkara, abhimana*) and the more their mind participates in the tranquility of the supramundane Reality, the less are their attachments to earthly joys and pleasures. The bliss of the Self is unexcelled, and in

comparision with it the pleasures of the world seem vain. To cite
the immortal words of Lord Krishna in the *Bhagavad-Gita*
(XVIII.37–39) once more:

> . . . that which in the beginning is like poison and with the
> changes [brought about in the course of time] becomes like
> nectar—that happiness (*sukha*) is called *sattva*-natured; it is
> born from the clear wisdom of the Self.

> That which [arises] through the union of the senses [with their
> corresponding] objects is like nectar in the beginning and with
> the changes [of time] becomes like poison—that happiness is
> regarded as *rajas*-natured.

> [That] happiness which in the beginning and in its sequel de-
> ludes the self, arising from sleep, slothfulness and negli-
> gence—that is designated as *tamas*-natured.

FIERY ASCETICISM

The third component of self-restraint is austerity, or *tapas*. This
word is derived from the root *tap* meaning "to burn, glow," and literally denotes "heat" or "glow." It stands for fiery asceticism or
fierce austerities. In the *Yoga-Bhashya* (II.32), the term is explained
as the ability to endure extremes such as heat and cold.

The metamorphosis attempted in mythic Yoga proceeds on the
basis of an explosive temporary intensification of consciousness
known as samadhi, or "ecstasy." These momentary switches of
consciousness are the result of most intense psychomental concentration. This can be accompanied by a marked rise in body temperature, especially when the *kundalini* process of Hatha-Yoga is
involved.

This phenomenon of psychosomatic heat has been given particular attention in Tibetan Tantrism where it forms the basis of a
specific yogic technique, called *gtum-mo* in the Tibetan language. It
is designed to produce such heat as a means of consciousness unification.

The practice of *tapas* is very ancient, and so are the philosophical or mythological ideas surrounding it. Thus, the Vedic Indians
related the phenomenon of psychosomatic heat to the great events

at the beginning of time. They thought that the world emerged from a primeval Person, who caused all creation through an act of self-heating (tapas). This old cosmogonic notion found its way into the *Brihad-Aranyaka-Upanishad* (I.2.6), the earliest esoteric Hindu scripture. Here we are told a profound mystery:

He desired: "Let me sacrifice again with a great sacrifice." He exerted himself. He practiced austerity. When he had exerted himself in austerity, his glory and vigor went forth. Glory and vigor, verily, are the life forces (*prana*). So when the life forces departed, his body began to swell . . .

It is instructive to compare this cosmogonic motif with the deliberate heating of ascetics, which has no other purpose than that of melting down their individual cosmos. In other words, the original act of creation is reversed. That which has flown out of the One through tapas is called back again by the same process. Symbolically speaking, the ascetic ordeal is a recapitulation on the microcosmic level of the primordial sacrifice, which the primal Person (*adi-purusha*) performed on himself in order to call the universe into existence.

Sacrifice and asceticism are closely related ideas and practices, and some ancient Sanskrit texts even speak of asceticism as the inner sacrifice.

Tapas is the appropriation and utilization of the powers inherent in the created universe, by which ascetics can attain to the autonomy of the primordial creator. They then gain supremacy over all beings and things and can, like Lord Shiva, destroy or save, curse or bless. Or, as the mythic Yoga demands, they can abandon their physical existence altogether and transcend the universe to reach identification with the supramundane One beyond all manifest realms.

Tapas comprises such practices as lengthy fasts, standing under the midday sun, sitting immobile, total concentration during the construction of the sacrificial altar, or prolonged breath retention while reciting the sacred lore. The *Mahabharata* epic contains numerous episodes in which such exercises are described and praised. For example, the twelfth book (XII.262ff.) relates the story of the merchant Tuladhara of Benares. He is said to have stood stock-still for many months in order not to disturb the birds who had built their nest on top of his head.

According to Patanjali the fruit of asceticism is the perfection of the body and its organs, which reaches its peak with the attainment of the magic powers (siddhi).[2] Furthermore, the body is said to become well-shaped, lovely, strong, and robust as a diamond.[3] The type of asceticism conducive to such desirable ends has obviously little in common with the useless and positively harmful self-castigation and self-mutilation resorted to by misled fakirs. No one is plainer about this than Lord Krishna, who in the *Bhagavad-Gita* (XVII.14–19) speaks about the three fundamental types of asceticism:

> Worship of the gods, the twice-born ones, the teachers and the wise, as well as purity, uprightness, chastity, and nonharming is called asceticism of the body.

> Speech that causes no disquiet, is truthful, pleasant, and beneficial, as well as the practice of self-study is called asceticism of speech.

> Serenity of mind, gentleness, silence, self-restraint, and purification of the [inner] states: this is called mental asceticism.

> This threefold asceticism practiced with supreme faith by men who are yoked and not longing for the fruit [of their deeds] is designated as *sattva*-natured.

> Asceticism that is performed for the sake of [obtaining] good treatment, honor, and reverence and with ostentation: this is called here [in this world] *rajas*-natured. It is fickle and unsteady.

> Asceticism that is performed with foolish conceptions [such as the aim] of torturing oneself or that has the purpose of ruining others: this is called *tamas*-natured.

Tapas must on no account degenerate into fakiristic self-torture, which only weakens the body-mind. On the contrary, it is meant to strengthen the physical frame and the mind and render both fully operational. As the *Maitrayaniya-Upanishad* (IV.3) announces:

> Through asceticism clarity (*sattva*) is attained; through clarity, the mind-essence (*manas*)[4] is attained; through the mind-essence, the Self is attained. He who has attained the Self does not return.

STUDY AS A PATHWAY TO THE SELF

The fourth practice of self-restraint is svadhyaya, or "self-study." Like asceticism, it is also an integral part of the ancient ritualism of the brahmins. The word itself is composed of *sva* ("own") and *adhyaya* (from *adhi* + *a* + *aya* = "to go into"), meaning "one's own going or delving into." It stands for the absorption into the sacred texts, which in Vedic times were studied either silently (in the village) or recited aloud (outside the village). The *Shata-Patha* ("Hundred Paths")-*Brahmana* (XI.5.7.I.), an early ritual text, contains a passage that vividly describes the extraordinary value attached to this particular discipline:

> The study and the interpretation [of the sacred scriptures] are [a source] of joy [for the serious student]. He becomes of yoked mind and independent of others, and day by day he gains [spiritual] power. He sleeps peacefully and is his own best physician. He controls the senses and delights in the One. His insight and [inner] glory grow, [and he obtains the ability] to influence the world.

Svadhyaya must not be confused with intellectual learning; rather it is the meditative recitation of, and absorption into, the ancient wisdom. It is the immersion into the vibration of the chanted words to which a special power is attributed. Through monotonous recitation (*japa*), the power of sound is unlocked and the mind of the reciter is transported into the center of the sacred words, where he or she becomes aware of their deep inner meaning. Hence we find that the illustrious Bhoja, the tenth-century ruler of Dhara, interpreted svadhyaya simply as the recitation of mantras. In the context of Classical Yoga, however, this amounts to an oversimplification. A more rounded understanding of self-study is expressed in the *Vishnu-Purana* (VI.6.2–3a):

> From self-study one should proceed to Yoga and from Yoga to self-study. By perfection in self-study and Yoga the supreme · Self becomes manifest. Study is one eye to behold that [Self], and Yoga is the other.

DEVOTION TO THE ARCH-YOGIN

One feature of self-restraint still remains to be discussed, which is *ishvara-pranidhana*, or devotion to the Lord. This element of the yogic path requires special attention, as it has always been either completely misinterpreted or rather underestimated in its practical significance.

According to Patanjali's Yoga aphorisms (I.24), the Lord (ishvara) is a special transcendental Self. He differs from the other Selves (purusha) insofar as he is eternally undefiled by the causes of suffering, by action and its fruit, as well as by the karmic deposits (*ashaya*) in the depth of the psyche. In other words, the Lord is without karma, just as he is without body-mind.

The other Selves, however, are liable to fall victim to the illusion that they are associated with a finite form. This illusion is the state of unenlightenment, or bondage, which has no beginning. There are simply countless numbers of beings in the world, who do not know their true status as the Self.

Yet, the Selves are never *really* deprived of their authentic nature. It only appears so from the viewpoint of the individual psyche. When we cease to identify with "our" body-mind, we awaken again as the transcendental Self.

In the philosophy of Classical Yoga, the Lord is neither the creator of the world, nor is he actively engaged in its sustenance or its destruction. For, according to Patanjali's cosmology, Nature (*prakriti*) is autonomous. Like the Phoenix of mythology, it consumes itself and rises from its own ashes *ad infinitum*.

The Awareness monads, or Selves, are eternally separated from this drama and only mistakenly believe themselves to have forfeited their intrinsic freedom. As soon as they reawaken to their essence, they realize that in truth they were never subject to the laws of Nature, but had simply been deceived by a mirage of their own making.

This clear-cut dualism between the Awareness monads and unconscious Nature is philosophically unconvincing. Such a conception springs from a one-sided rationalistic approach, and we may speculate that this metaphysical dualism was the main reason for the lack of success of Patanjali's Yoga as an independent philosophical system.

Although it was logical for Patanjali to place the Lord on the side of the Selves rather than that of insentient Nature, his model nevertheless seems rather contrived. This has prompted some critics to regard the theistic element in Classical Yoga as an altogether foreign substance. However, the assertion that the ishvara has found his way surreptitiously into the dualistic ontology of Patanjali's model is unwarranted. For, it overlooks the fact that grace (*prasada*), as embodied in the concept of the Lord, has been an integral element of the yogic tradition from earliest times. Already the Vedic priests understood their states of absorption as "god-given."[5]

Nonetheless, it is quite correct, as one scholar observed, that the practice of devotion to the Lord "can hardly be called a genuine devotion, since its sole purpose is not a submission to God, not an attitude of love and adoration, but only to 'attain singleness of intent.'"[6] Still, it is definitely wrong to think that "one could very well cut out the sutras relating to the Lord, without even leaving a trace of excision."[7]

The popular academic notion that the conception of God was interpolated into Classical Yoga is completely unfounded. Nor is it tenable to reduce God to a mere archetype of the yogin, as for example Mircea Eliade suggested.[8] Neither can the fact that Patanjali retained the theistic conception be explained away as a simple concession to the vital panentheistic tradition of Yoga. Instead we ought to seriously consider the possibility that Patanjali's firm adherence to theism could well have its roots in the actual inner experiences of yogins.

What does the practice of devotion to the Lord entail? Vyasa, on the whole the most reliable commentator on the *Yoga-Sutra*, furnishes some very useful observations:

On account of devotion [to the Lord], [that is] through a particular love-attachment (*bhakti*) [to him], the Lord inclines [toward the yogin] and favors him alone by reason of his [meditative and devotional] disposition. By this disposition only, the yogin draws near to the attainment of ecstasy and to the fruit of ecstasy [which is emancipation].[9]

This statement only allows for the psychic component of the devotion to the Lord, which is the disposition of loving reorientation of the mind to God. Vyasa therefore supplements it by the following remark:

Devotion to the Lord is the offering-up of all deeds to the supreme Teacher, or the renunciation of their fruits.[10]

With this explanation, Vyasa quite obviously takes up the fundamental doctrine of the *Bhagavad-Gita* that spiritual practitioners have to conceive and experience their every action and thought as a sacrifice proffered to the supreme Being. However narrow and unacceptable the conception of God in Classical Yoga may appear, the devotional element in it can neither be ignored nor denied. The yogic work is always sacred and consecrating. Although the Lord is formally differentiated from the countless Self-monads, we must assume that on that absolute level of existence he fully coincides with them. In other words, there is only a numerical multiplicity. Qualitatively, the Lord and the Self-monads are one; for all Selves are omnipresent and hence intersect in eternity.

This is also the conclusion reached by Shankara in his recently discovered commentary on the *Yoga-Sutra*. Likewise, the modern yogin and scholar Hariharananda noted in his *Yoga-Bhasvati* (I.24):

All the "Seers" [i.e., transcendental Selves] freed from consciousness, are of one nature, and on account of this interfusion there is no way of telling them apart.

NOTES

1. Swami Sivananda, *Practice of Yoga* (Sivanandanagar, India: Yoga-Vedanta Forest Academy Press, 1970), pp. 68–69.

2. See *Yoga-Sutra* III.45.

3. See *Yoga-Sutra* III.46.

4. The word *manas*, which usually stands for the lower mind, is here translated as "mind-essence," because obviously a higher cognitive faculty is intended. Probably, in this context, *manas* signifies what elsewhere is the function of *buddhi*, the faculty of higher intelligence.

5. See, for example, *Rig-Veda* I.37.4 and VIII.32.27.

6. G.M. Koelman, *Patanjala Yoga* (Poona: Papal Atheneum, 1970), p. 58.

7. *Ibid.*, p. 58.

8. M. Eliade, *Yoga: Immortality and Freedom* (Princeton, NJ: Princeton University Press, 1970), p. 73ff.

9. *Yoga-Bhashya* I.23.

10. *Yoga-Bhashya* II.I. See also II.32.

CHAPTER 15

THE IMMOBILIZED BODY

POSTURE AS SACRAMENT

Our Western habit of sitting on specially manufactured furniture is characteristic of our estrangement from Nature. In contrast, the squatting position assumed by members of traditional societies portrays their much closer psychic connection to the soil. Our sitting elevated on chairs and couches is neither the authority-conscious throning of the priest or heaven-inspired king nor the unassuming, close-to-nature cowering of the Indian, African, or Arab peasant.

Strictly speaking, our way of sitting, usually with slouched shoulders, is simply a false bodily attitude. So is the stiff sitting with upright spine and legs neatly positioned close together on formal occasions. Both postures suggest inner tension and a certain lack of grace. In other words, our Western-style sitting faithfully reflects the decadence of our postindustrial civilization.

Yogins know a special kind of sitting, a throning without throne. They remain close to the soil, yet they do not cower in peasant fashion. Rather, their whole bodily poise indicates their spiritual transcendence of Nature. Neither do they sit in the rigidly hieratic manner of a pharaoh or Mayan god-king, who saw themselves as representatives, or marionettes, of higher powers.

The special yogic way of sitting is the *asana*. This Sanskrit word is composed of the verbal root *as* "to sit" and the neuter ending *ana*. In the asana, or yogic posture, the body itself is made an instrument of elevation. Just as our sitting on chairs inhibits the body-mind and prevents it from unfolding its inner potential, so the asana opens up a pathway to inwardness and the spiritual dimension.

The asana is not a purely physical exercise, although it is often treated as such by Western Yoga students, who "do" their daily routine. The yogic posture is a sacramental act. It is assumed with a distinct inner disposition, marked by relaxed vigilance and peace.

The asana is assumed by bringing the extremities closer to the bodily axis. The legs are folded so as to form a stable platform for the rest of the body, while the dangling arms are brought together to create a closed circuit. In this way the body is rendered homogeneous. Symbolically speaking, the yogic posture is the assimilation of the spinal column to the world axis, Mount Meru. The body is thus rendered into a sacred place.

This is an important phase in the process of directing the consciousness inward. Without the somatic homogeneity created by the asana, no real inner focusing or openness to the transcendental Being is possible. By means of the asana, practitioners awaken to the intrinsic aliveness of the body, experiencing it as a field of energy rather than a solid form. Historian of religion Mircea Eliade proffered these illuminating comments:

> *Asana* is distinctly a sign of transcending the human condition. . . . What is certain is that the motionless, hieratic position of the body imitates some other condition than the human; the yogin in the state of asana can be homologized with a plant or a sacred statue; under no circumstances can he be homologized with man qua man, who, by definition, is mobile, restless, agitated, unrhythmic.[1]

Eliade went on to say that the asana is to the body what concentration is to the mind. The body is focused, immobilized, and made single. He rightly described the asana as an "archetypal, iconographic posture."

What the asana is in a technical sense can be expressed in the following formula:

Asana = steady bodily posture + relaxedness (*shaithilya*) +
         coinciding with the infinite consciousness-ether.

This definition is derived from two of Patanjali's aphorisms (II.46 and 48), which read:

The posture [must be] steady and pleasant.—[It comes about] through the relaxation of tensions and by coinciding with the infinite [consciousness-ether].

The first part of this stipulation is self-explanatory. Without stability, the posture would hardly serve yogins in their task. Furthermore, if it were uncomfortable it would merely interfere with the inner work. On the contrary, when properly accomplished, the posture is comfortable and pleasant. It is accompanied by the relaxation of muscular tension as well as mental tension.

The curious phrase "coinciding with the infinite" (*ananta-samapatti*) can be explained as signifying the feeling of expansion that occurs in deep relaxation. The classical commentators understood the word "infinite" (*ananta*) as a proper name, taking it to refer to the mythological serpent-king whose infinite body serves God Vishnu as a couch. Ananta, or Shesha, is a symbol of infinity and power.

However, Patanjali himself may have had a different, nonmythological explanation in mind. Ananta could also simply stand for the infinite inner space, which opens up when consciousness is withdrawn from external objects. During the asana, the body loses its rigid form and is experienced as a quivering force field charged with life.

This also explains why the yogic posture is said to make the practitioner insensitive to the pairs of opposites, such as heat and cold, silence and noise, light and darkness, and so on. The asana contains an element of sensory inhibition. It is a first stepping-stone in the process of meditative absorption.

THE LONG HISTORY OF SACRAMENTAL POSTURES

The asanas have their historical root in the trance postures of ancient Shamanism. As anthropologist Felicitas Goodman has shown, shamans around the world have used a limited number of bodily attitudes to facilitate their vision quest.[2] Apparently certain postures, combined with rhythmic drumming, can induce an altered state of consciousness even in ordinary people. Moreover, each posture seems to correspond to a different inner state. This is also the experience of Yoga practitioners in regard to the postures

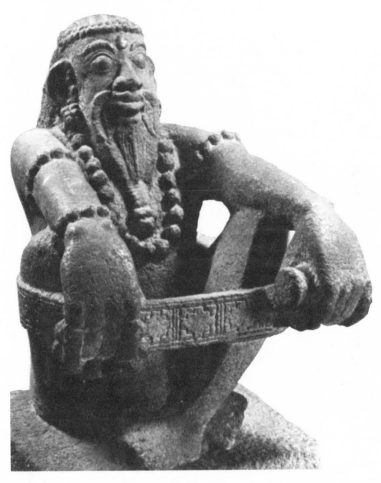

*Seventeenth-century Hindu sculpture of yogin sitting
cross-legged with the aid of a knee band.
Victoria and Albert Museum, London.*

known as *mudras* or "gestures." Particularly sensitive practitioners are able to detect subtle psychic changes in connection with the regular asanas as well.

Depictions of yoga-like sitting positions have been found on steatite seals unearthed in the great cities of the Indus civilization. On one seal, some scholars believe they recognize the later god Shiva, lord of the yogins and master of wild beasts. However, this interpretation is uncertain.[3] Our knowledge of this mysterious civilization, which collapsed about 1800 B.C., is still rather incomplete. Nor are we likely to find definite answers to this and many other riddles until the hieroglyphic script has been deciphered.

Be that as it may, there can be no doubt at all that the typical asana is very old. The word itself first appears in the 2,800-year-old *Brihad-Aranyaka-Upanishad* (VI.2.4) and the equally ancient *Taittiriya-Upanishad* (I.II.3). In both scriptures, however, the term is still used in the sense of "seat" or "platform." This is also the meaning of the word as it occurs in the *Bhagavad-Gita* (VI.11–14):

> Setting up a steady seat for himself in a pure place, neither too high nor too low, with a cloth, deer-skin or grass upon it, there making the mind one-pointed, restraining the activity of mind and senses, he should, seated on the seat, yoke himself in Yoga for the purification of the self.
>
> Equable, keeping trunk, head and neck motionless and steady, gazing [relaxedly] at the tip of the nose, without looking round about him, with tranquil self and devoid of fear, steadfast in the vow of celibacy, controlling the mind, thoughts on Me, [fully] yoked—he should sit, intent on Me.

It is hard to guess at what moment in time the term asana assumed the meaning of "posture." The first important occurrence is in the *Yoga-Sutra*, which must be placed in the second or third century A.D. Here the term is clearly defined. Then, in the mid-fifth century, Vyasa mentions a great variety of yogic postures in his celebrated commentary on the Yoga aphorisms. Among the asanas he mentions are the lotus posture (*padma-asana*), the heroic posture (*vira-*), the auspicious posture (*bhadra-*), the staff posture (*danda-*) and the *svastika* posture.[4] Vyasa also speaks of certain "seats" (*nishadana*) named after animals and of the *paryanka* or "couch" posture, which was the favorite of the Buddha. Furthermore, he refers to a posture for which a "support" is used, which Vacaspati Mishra specifies as a yogic table (*yoga-pattaka*). Evidently Vyasa only mentioned some of the postures known and practiced during his time.

The golden season of the yogic postures, however, comes only with the emergence of Tantric Yoga, particularly Hatha-Yoga and the *kaya-sadhana* movement which sought Self-realization through the proper employment of the body. According to the Hatha-Yoga texts, there are as many postures as there are living beings and the symbolic figure 8,400,000 is frequently mentioned in this context. Of these only eighty-four postures are supposed to be useful, of which again only thirty-two are said to be particularly suited for human beings.

Originally asanas were purely meditational postures and only with the Tantric revolution did they receive a completely new purpose, when the asana became an instrument for the perfection of the body. This positive conception is foreign to mythic Yoga for which as in Orphism the body represents only the "tomb" of the soul.

NOTES

1. M. Eliade, *Yoga: Immortality and Freedom* (Princeton, NJ: Princeton University Press, 1970), p. 54.

2. See F. D. Goodman, *Where the Spirits Ride the Wind: Trance Journeys and Other Ecstatic Experiences* (Bloomington and Indianapolis, IN: Indiana University Press, 1990).

3. See, for example, the critical remarks by H.P. Sullivan, "A reexamination of the religion of the Indus civilization," *History of Religions*, vol. 4, no. 1 (Chicago, 1964), pp. 118ff.

4. See *Yoga-Bhashya* II.46.

CHAPTER 16

THE TRANSFORMATIVE FUNCTION OF THE BREATH

THE ESOTERIC TEACHING ABOUT THE LIFE FORCE

The process of psychosomatic transformation and energization initiated with the practice of bodily posture is continued and enhanced through the regulation of the life force (prana), which is the fourth limb of the eightfold path taught by Patanjali.

The technical term for this practice is *pranayama*, which is commonly translated as "breath control." However, this rendering is somewhat imprecise because prana does not merely refer to the breath but to the underlying life force. The physiological activity of breathing is only the external aspect of the subtle movement of prana.

The life force is thought to interpenetrate the entire universe and to function as a kind of *élan vital*. It is, as the *Yoga-Vasishtha* (III.13.31) puts it, "vibratory force" (*spanda-shakti*). Although speculations about this all-pervading energy reach as far back as the time of the *Atharva-Veda* (XV), none of the classical Sanskrit works seems to contain a satisfactory definition of this important concept. When we assemble the various statements found in the Hindu scriptures, we arrive at the following understanding.

Prana is an effluence or aspect of the transcendental Being. It is neither air, nor is it identical with sensory activity, but is the common foundation of both. It is the material out of which the subtle body (*sukshma-sharira*) is built. This energy body is known in the Western occult tradition as the "astral body," "etheric body," or "double."

Although a homogeneous force, prana assumes a fivefold appearance in the human body or rather its subtle counterpart. As *prana* it draws life force into the body; on the physical level this appears as inhalation. As *apana*, corresponding to exhalation, it releases the life force from the body. In the form of *vyana* it circulates through the whole body. As *samana* it effects mainly the assimilation of food, and as *udana* it is the uprising vital force that is especially responsible for the separation of the subtle body from the physical vehicle at death.

In the ancient *Chandogya-Upanishad* (II.13.6), these five forms of the life energy are called the "gate keepers to the heavenly world," and only those who know their secret can hope to reach the Absolute. It is particularly the cyclic activity of prana (manifesting as inhalation) and apana (manifesting as exhalation) which the yogin must fully understand and master. The *Goraksha-Samhita* (I.38–40), one of the older Hatha-Yoga texts, has these explanatory stanzas:

> As a ball hit with a crook flies up, so consciousness (*jiva*), propelled by *prana* and *apana*, does not stand still.

> Under the impact of *prana* and *apana*, consciousness rushes up and down through the left and right pathways, and because of this fickleness it cannot be perceived.

> As a hawk tied to a rope can be brought back again [when it has] flown away, so consciousness bound to the constituents (*guna*) [of Nature] is pulled along by *prana* and *apana*.

To comprehend the full meaning of this passage, it must be read in conjunction with a parallel explanation in the *Yoga-Shikha-Upanishad* (59–60):

> Consciousness (*citta*) is connected with the vital force indwelling in all beings. Like a bird tied to a string: so is this mind.

> The mind is not brought under control by many considerations. The [only] means for its control is nothing else but the life force.

UNIFICATION THROUGH BREATH CONTROL

It is this discovery of the mutual dependence of consciousness and life force that has led to the invention of special breathing practices by which it is possible to influence the mind. The main purpose of these practices is to change the ordinarily irregular flow of the vital energy by bringing it under conscious control. This adjustment of prana is followed by a gradual expansion of its cyclic movement.

On the physical level this entails a progressive lengthening of the period of breath retention. According to the *Amara-Kosha*, a Sanskrit dictionary of the fifth century A.D., this dilation of the breath is the exact meaning of the word *ayama* in pranayama.[1] Breath retention is the "nuts and bolts" of yogins and ascetics, and occasionally their enthusiasm for this practice has led to gross exaggerations. The Indian scholar Surendra Nath Dasgupta made the following pertinent comments:

> At first the breath that is taken in is kept perhaps for a few minutes and then slowly exhaled. The practice is continued for days and months, the period of the retention of the breath taken in being gradually increased. With the growth of breath-control, one may keep his breath suspended, without exhalation or inhalation, for hours, days, months and even years together. With the suspension of the respiratory process the body remains in a state of suspended animation, without any external signs of life. The heart ceases to beat, there is neither taking in of food nor evacuation of any sort, there is no movement of the body. . . . Even in modern times there are many well-attested cases of yogis who can remain in this apparently lifeless condition for more than a month. I have myself seen a case where the yogi stayed in this condition for nine days.[2]

Fascinating as such cases are, they must be regarded as regrettable deviations. In Yoga proper, breath control has an altogether different purpose. The slowing-down of respiration, which is accompanied by the elimination of external stimuli, results in an immediate intensification of consciousness. Normally, breathing is irregular and shallow; it backs up the discontinuity of the profane mind, as is evident from the constantly changing degree and focus of attention, the unsteady flow of thoughts, as well as the fluctuating emotional disposition.

Through the practice of prana regulation, a state of inner balance is achieved that creates the inner continuum necessary

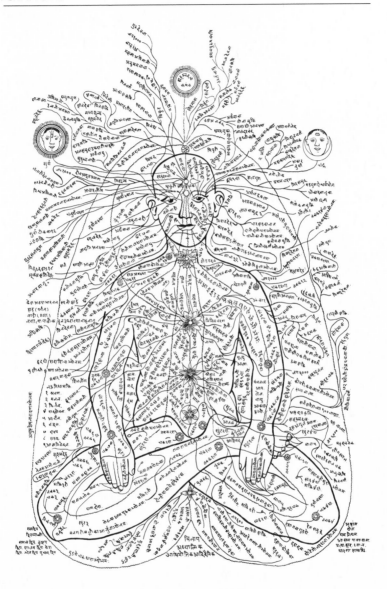

Human body showing the currents of life energy (prana), with major vortices (cakra).

for full-fledged meditation. As King Bhoja, a practicing yogin, summed it up in his *Raja-Martanda* (I.43):

> The triple control of the life force, [consisting in] the phase of injection, expulsion and retention, binds consciousness to [a fixed] area by way of one-pointedness and owing to the priority of the *prana* activity [in relation to] all sense activity, as well as because of the coordination [that exists between] operation and inactivity of mind and life force in their respective functions. The suppressed life force effects the one-pointedness of consciousness by means of the restriction of the entire sense activity, and it causes the host of defects (*dosha*) to dwindle, as we hear in the scriptures. And [let us recall that] all distracting [mental] activity is caused by the defects.

The defects spoken of here are the five undesirable psychomental states frequently named in the Yoga literature as passion, delusion, attachment, desire, and anger. However, various schools mention different sets of these inauspicious mental conditions. Some also list sleep and faulty breathing, others greed, envy, and pride. All these correspond roughly to the Christian notion of the "seven deadly sins" or *peccata capitalia*, namely pride, avarice, lechery, envy, gluttony, anger, and sloth.

These inauspicious states, King Bhoja assures us, can all be overcome by controlling the life force within the body. They are overcome simply because attention is subtracted from the external world and its multiple enticements.

In Hatha-Yoga, many techniques are employed to gain mastery over the breath. Most important, however, are those practices that enable the ascetic to prolong the period of what is called the "pot" (*kumbhaka*). This refers to breath retention either after inhaling or after exhaling. The idea is to acquire such control that the flow of the life force in the body can be consciously directed along the spinal axis toward the crown of the head and into the space beyond.

When the life force is confined within the body, this creates a highly charged psychosomatic condition, which is accompanied by certain physical symptoms, notably a rise in body temperature.

The ascetics use this compressed energy to catapult themselves, in consciousness, beyond the boundaries of the body into the state of deep concentration and meditation.

At the highest stage of accomplishment in breath control, the practitioner is said to be able to levitate. Whether true or not, this epitomizes the great hope of the mythic traditions to leave the solid ground and ascend to the Self.

The world-transcending thrust of mythic spirituality can also be seen in the following quotation from the *Hatha-Ratna-Vali* (III.98):

> The yogin who is accomplished in controlling the life force is like [God] Vishnu or the Great Lord. That yogin is all the gods. [Therefore] he should not be slighted.

In other words, the masters of breath control are no longer ordinary mortals. They are superbeings, deities who do not belong to this material universe. Gods like Vishnu or Shiva are yogic archetypes. They are the true masters of the life force. The adepts who know the secrets of the prana current are said to be their equals.

NOTES

1. The term *pranayama* is composed of *prana* and *ayama*. In Sanskrit when a word ending in "a" is joined with a word beginning with "a," the result is a long "a." Publications using a more scholarly nomenclature indicate this by the letter "ā".

2. S. Dasgupta, *Hindu Mysticism* (Chicago: Chicago University Press, 1927), p. 75.

CHAPTER 17

THE TORTOISE-LIKE WITHDRAWAL OF ATTENTION

THE VICIOUS CYCLE OF SENSORY INVOLVEMENT

The regulation of the life force by means of the breath, as we have seen, creates a great aggregation of psychosomatic energy. This, in turn, facilitates enhanced mental concentration. However, this gain in energy and mental focus is traded off for reduced sensory feedback. Attention can look either outward toward the sensible world or inward, and each direction has its own distinct set of psychosomatic characteristics.

At any rate, ascetics who aspire to transcend the body-mind welcome the decreased sensitivity to sensory stimuli that accompanies the process of introversion. As the mind is turned inward on itself, the external reality is progressively shut out. Finally a state is reached in which consciousness is completely internalized and in a way hermetically sealed off from the outer world. It can then no longer be distracted by any sensory information.

The German psychiatrist J.H. Schultz, inventor of the Autogenic Training, which has been called the Western equivalent of Yoga, once defined this process as the "subtraction" of the psychic energies from external events.[1] The corresponding Sanskrit terms are *pratyahara* or *pratyahriti*, both of which mean "drawing back" or "withdrawal."

A favorite picture used in the Sanskrit scriptures to describe this gradual withdrawal from the sense objects is that of a tortoise retracting its limbs. In the more scholastic language of Patanjali, pratyahara is "a disjunction of the senses from their respective objects [and] an imitation as it were of the nature of consciousness.[2] That is to say, sensory inhibition seeks to establish consciousness in itself, without its usual flux toward the external reality.

The feedback from the senses constantly entices us to project our consciousness outward by an act of attention. This trajectory of the mind, however, holds no promise for ascetics who believe that the outer world is merely an abode of suffering. For them, the senses are in the service of karma. They ensure that the wheel of existence continues to whirl, grinding all beings to dust.

The senses are likened to unruly horses that draw the chariot, the mind, aimlessly hither and tither. Hence, as the *Mahabharata* (XII.249.3) states, they must be controlled "as a father keeps a tight rein on his sons." The fatal consequence of unbridled sense activity is aptly portrayed in the *Bhagavad-Gita* (II.62–63):

When a man absorbs himself in the sense objects, contact is born to them. From contact springs desire; from desire anger is bred.

From anger comes bewilderment; from bewilderment, disorder of the memory; from disorder of the memory, the destruction of [higher] understanding (*buddhi*). Upon the destruction of [higher] understanding, one is lost.

The above verses summarize very dramatically the vicious cycle in which ordinary worldlings are entrapped. The starting-point of it all is the body's natural tendency to receive the world into itself via the senses. So, for the yogins this is also the place where the most stringent control must be exercised. The lever of control is obviously consciousness itself. As Vyasa explained in his *Yoga-Bhashya* (II.54):

Just as when the queen-bee flies up and the bees swarm after her and when she settles down [the bees also] settle, so the senses are controlled when consciousness (*citta*) is controlled.

Sensory inhibition and the centralization of consciousness are a synchronous process. The anonymous author of the *Katha-Upanishad* (VI.10–11), who lived in the fifth century B.C., put it this way:

When the five [sense] functions together with the mind are at rest and the wisdom-faculty (*buddhi*) does not stir—this, they say, is the supreme course.

This they consider to be Yoga: the firm holding back of the

senses. Then one becomes undistracted. Yoga, truly, is a beginning and an end.[3]

Yoga is a beginning and an end because, on the one side, it discontinues our sensory involvement with the world and, on the
other side, it opens up the inner world and also that which transcends consciousness.

SELF-REALIZATION THROUGH SENSORY SHUT-DOWN

The world of objects is shunned because in mythic spirituality
it is thought to block access to the Self, which is the ultimate good.
Our true essence can only be found within, and the senses are incapable of reaching it. Only complete inner stillness can give birth to
that ineffable state of realization in which Being-Awareness shines
forth in its undiluted splendor. As the *Mahabharata* epic declares:

> The Self (*atman*) cannot be perceived with the senses which
> disunited scatter to and fro and are difficult to restrain for
> those whose self is not prepared. (XII.194.58)

> Clinging to that [ultimate Reality], the sage should, through
> absorption, concentrate his mind to one point by "clenching"
> the host of senses and sitting like a log.

> He should not perceive sound with his ear, not feel touch with
> his skin. He should not perceive form with his eye and not
> taste tastes with his tongue.

> Also, the knower of Yoga should, through absorption, abstain
> from all smells. He should courageously reject these agitators
> of the group of five [senses]. (XII.195.5–7)

However, withdrawal of the senses is only really possible
when the ascetics have also succeeded in gaining inner distance
from mundane things. In other words, an act of will alone is not
enough to curb the senses. They must also enjoy a deep inner im-
munity against the fascinations of life. Above all, they must be
firmly set on the realization of the Self. If this is not true of them,
they are apt to fail in disconnecting their consciousness from the
world of objects. Perhaps they will succeed temporarily, but before

long their unresolved desires will cast them out of the state of inner balance.

Sensory abstraction is thus an integral part of the great *Via negativa* of mythic spirituality, the path of negation of the manifest universe. By means of sense-withdrawal, the ascetics seek to de-condition the mind and realign it to a higher purpose.

There is one final point that merits emphasis, namely the fact that the regulation of the life force through breathing techniques and the practice of sense-withdrawal, as well as the resulting state of meditative absorption are all phases of one and the same process of interiorization. The following stanzas from the *Bhagavad-Gita* (V.27–28) illustrate this continuity perfectly:

> Shutting out [all] external contacts and [fixing] the sight between the eyebrows, making even the in-flow and out-flow [of the life force in the form of breath] moving within the nostrils, that sage whose senses, mind and wisdom-faculty are controlled is [soon] truly liberated.

That the practices of breath control, sense-withdrawal, concentration, and meditation are in fact continuous phases rather than isolated stages is also corroborated by the fact that in some schools, breath control is listed after sense-withdrawal. In practice, both promote each other, and together they unify and transform the consciousness of the yogin.

NOTES

1. See J.H. Schultz, *Das Autogene Training: Konzentrative Selbstentspannung* (Leipzig: Thieme, 1940).

2. *Yoga-Sutra* II.54.

3. The Sanskrit phrase *yogo hi prabhava-apyayau* has been translated differently by interpreters of this ancient *Upanishad*. Some understand it as meaning "because Yoga can be acquired and lost." However, this does not really tally with the intent of the immediately preceding sentences. The interpretation adopted by the present author takes its lead from the *Mandukya-Upanishad* (6) where the phrase *prabhava-apyayau hi bhutanam* is found. It means "the origin and destination of beings" and here refers to the Lord of all.

CHAPTER 18

THE ONE-POINTED
CONSCIOUSNESS

IMMOBILIZATION OF THE MIND

In the *Mahabharata* epic (XII.306.16), which contains many intriguing passages of spiritual instruction, we find the following statement:

> When the yogin has successfully accomplished the withdrawal of the senses from their respective objects, then he does not hear, nor smell, nor taste, nor see, nor does he sense touch, and his mind no longer conceptualizes.

To what extent mental one-pointedness blocks out sense perceptions is exemplified in a story told about Mahavira, the founder of historical Jainism. While he was in a state of deep concentration, hooligans molested him with cruel tricks. They pierced his ears, pulled his hair, lacerated his skin, and even lit a fire between his feet. However, their barbaric acts completely failed to distract that great ascetic. Similarly, Mahavira's distinguished contemporary Gautama the Buddha is reported not to have heard the deafening bang accompanying the lightning that struck the ground near where he was steeped in meditation.

Accomplishment in the practice of sense-withdrawal renders the ascetics or yogins independent of the external world. This permits them to dedicate their attention fully to the inner reality and to proceed toward ever greater unification, until only the singular Being, the Self, shines forth.

This internal progression from the multitudinous mental contents to the one Being-Awareness occurs in three essential phases, namely concentration (dharana), meditative absorption (dhyana), and ecstasy (samadhi). These three limbs of the eightfold path of Classical Yoga are collectively referred to as the "inner limbs," as opposed to the previous five "outer limbs," comprising moral discipline, self-restraint, posture, regulation of the life force, and sensory inhibition.

What is concentration in this context? The most precise definition is given in the *Yoga-Sutra* (III.1), which typifies it as "the binding of consciousness to [a single] place." In his Sanskrit commentary on this work, Vyasa comments as follows:

> Concentration is the binding of consciousness—merely [in the form of its] fluctuations—to the navel center, the lotus of the heart, the light in the head, the tip of the nose, the tip of the tongue or similar places, or to an external object.[1]

In modern parlance, the phrase "binding of consciousness" denotes the fixation of attention. The mind is made concentric with a particular mental object. Vyasa's statement received further elaboration at the hands of the renowned ninth-century scholar Vacaspati Mishra, who observed:

> On this there is also [a fitting reference] in the [*Vishnu-*] *Purana* (VI.7.45): "After the 'wind' [i.e., the life force] is controlled through the regulation of *prana* and the senses through sense-withdrawal, [the yogin] should let his consciousness rest on an appropriate 'prop'." Suitable external props are [the iconographic images of] Hiranyagarbha, Vasava, Prajapati, and so on.[2]

Of course, even these so-called external props are duly internalized. Concentration can only be practiced in regard to a mental image, whether it derives from the realm of phantasy or the world of objects. Thus, the practitioners focus on their image or idea of a particular deity, not the deity itself, although their concentration is said to bring them into contact with the deity itself. The reason for this is the parallelism that exists between the microcosm and the macrocosm. Our thoughts are ways of getting in touch with reality.

Thus, when we think of Shiva, Vishnu, Brahma, or the Self, we do not merely remain locked into our nervous system or brain. We also come into contact with those realities. Hence many authorities recommend that it profits one to focus on the very highest reality, which is the transcendental Self itself. Although the Self is always said to be beyond all conception, it is nevertheless by our intention that we can align ourselves with it.

Indeed, without this correspondence between thought and reality, all spiritual paths would be entirely superfluous. The power of thought, or the right deployment of attention, is the most profound secret of the spiritual traditions.

In the *Trishikhi-Brahmana-Upanishad* (31), a medieval scripture, the unification of consciousness is described in these words: "Know concentration to be the holding of consciousness in an immovable state." It is, in other words, fixed attention, an asana of the mind. A favorite simile is that of the yogin as an archer whose target is the transcendental center within himself.[3] In narrowing his field of attention to a single spot, he effects, given sufficient intensity, a sudden rupture in the structure of the ordinary consciousness. This results in the desired breakthrough to the supraconscious clarity of the transcendental Being-Awareness. As the *Mahabharata* (XII.205.14) puts it:

> Closing all the gates [of the body], abiding in the mind and achieving one-pointedness in the mind, one attains to that Supreme [Being].

This focusing of consciousness also bears the technical name of "one-pointedness" (*eka-agrata*). Just how pointed concentration must be in order to effect a profound switch in consciousness is borne out by a story found in the *Katha-Sarit-Sagara* (VI.27). This work, which is a compilation of popular tales of all kinds, was authored by Somadeva, who lived in the eleventh century. The story goes as follows.

Vitastadatta was a merchant who had become converted to Buddhism. His son, in utter disdain, persisted in calling him immoral and irreligious. Vitastadatta felt outraged and brought the matter before the king. He promptly ordered the boy's execution at the end of a period of two months, entrusting him, until then, to the custody of his father. Brooding on his fate, the lad could neither eat nor sleep.

At the appointed time, the boy was again brought to the royal palace. Seeing his terror, the king addressed him thus: "Just as you fear death today, so are other beings equally afraid of death. Consequently, what higher aspiration could there be than that of practicing the Buddhist virtue of nonharming at all times, which preserves all creatures from such fear?"

The boy, by now deeply repentant, desired to be put on the path to right knowledge and salvation. Recognizing his sincerity, the king decided to initiate him by means of a test. He had a vessel brought to him, filled to the brim with oil, and ordered the youth to carry it around the city without spilling a drop of it, or else he would be executed on the spot. Glad of this chance to live, the boy was determined to succeed. Undaunted he looked neither right nor left, thinking only of the vessel in his hands, and returned at last to the king without having spilled a drop.

Knowing that a festival was in progress in the city, the king inquired whether the boy had seen anyone at all on the roads. The youth replied that he had heard and seen nothing. The king seemed pleased, spared his life, and admonished him to pursue the supreme goal of salvation with the same single-mindedness and ardor.

In order for attention to eliminate all the disturbing fluctuations within consciousness, it must be focused in laser-beam fashion. In the *Kshurika-Upanishad*, a more traditional metaphor is used, which compares concentration to a knife with which all knots of the body-mind are severed to free the Spirit. This medieval Yoga scripture prescribes a fascinating method that combines concentration with breath retention. The yogins are asked to "cut off" the one hundred "channels" through which the life force flows. In other words, they should gradually withdraw their consciousness from the different parts of the body and focus exclusively on the central channel called *sushumna* ("most gracious").

This axial channel runs straight to the crown of the head, which is the hidden gate to the Absolute. When the laserlike consciousness, energized by the gathered life force, moves up into and through that psychic doorway, it merges or realizes itself to be one with the infinite Spirit. In the words of the *Kshurika-Upanishad* (22–23):

As a swan, having cut through the fetters, flies straight up into the sky—so the psyche, having severed its bonds, always crosses over [the ocean of conditioned] existence.

As a lamp, at the moment of [the flame's] extinction, having burned up [all its fuel], ceases to function—thus the yogin, having burned out all karma, ceases to exist [as an individual separate from all other beings].

DANGERS ON THE PATH TO SINGLE-MINDEDNESS

The practice of concentration is by no means easy, for "thoughts are more numerous than grass." Neither is it foolproof. This is brought home in the *Mahabharata* (XII.300.54.5), which states:

It is possible to stand on the sharpened edge of a knife, but it is difficult for an unprepared psyche to stand in the concentrations of Yoga.

Miscarried concentrations, O friend, do not lead men to an auspicious goal, [but they are] like a vessel at sea without a captain.

The *Yoga-Sutra* (I.30) enumerates nine obstacles that can arise in the attempt to pacify the inner world. These are illness, languor, doubt, heedlessness, slothfulness, dissipation, wrong views, the inability to reach the various states of absorption, and the inability to remain in these states. As Patanjali explains in the immediately following aphorism (I.31), these are accompanied by pain, dejection, trembling of the body, and faulty inhalation and exhalation.

The importance of a perpetual guarding of consciousness is very vividly brought out in Shankara's popular didactic work *Viveka-Cudamani* (325):

When consciousness even slightly deviates from the goal and is directed outward, then it sinks, just as an accidentally dropped ball rolls down a flight of stairs.

We can readily appreciate that exercises in concentration alone do not suffice to control the mind. We may be able to suspend our thoughts temporarily, but they would soon bubble up again from the undercurrents deep within the psyche. Then our attention would attach itself to this or that emotion or unresolved conflict stored in the subconscious. Hence the need for all-round vigilance emphasized by all the great spiritual teachers.

The yogins are expected to be able not only to focus the mind for a limited period of time but to be in control of it also during the day, and even during dream sleep. Success in the practice of concentration thus depends on a pure and virtuous lifestyle. Spiritual life cannot be compartmentalized; it is a matter of the whole person. As we have seen, in mythic spirituality the path to the Self is founded on a total reversal of conventional values and attitudes. Concentration is only a reflection of a much broader centering process, which guides the practitioner to the Reality beyond space-time and its scattered objects.

NOTES

1. *Yoga-Bhashya* III.1.

2. *Tattva-Vaisharadi* III.1.

3. See, e.g., *Mahabharata* (XII.300.31) and *Mundaka-Upanishad* (II.3–4).

CHAPTER 19

THE VERTICAL PATH OF ABSORPTION

MEDITATION AS PROGRESSIVE MENTAL DECONDITIONING

Mythic spirituality is concerned with the ascent of consciousness toward the ultimate Reality. Meditation is a very important link in this endeavor. As the *Vedanta-Paribhasha* (8), a respected Sanskrit manual of nondualist metaphysics, states: "Meditation is the immediate cause of the realization of the Absolute." It is meditation that lifts the inner veils that prevent us from facing Reality in its nakedness.

If we compare concentration to a point, meditative absorption may be considered as its linear continuation. The object that is held in the act of concentration is now brought into full focus until it fills the entire space of consciousness. The *Yoga-Sutra* (III.2) defines this stage as "the continuity of ideas (*pratyaya*) in that [state of concentration]." A very similar definition is found in the *Vedanta-Sara* (192), which is a popular work on nondualism composed by the fifteenth-century Vedanta teacher Sadananda Yogendra. This text defines meditative absorption, here called *nididhyasana*, as "the flow of ideas consistent with the nondual Reality to the exclusion of inconsistent ideas such as the body, etc."

What does this mean? The German Yoga researcher J.W. Hauer, who acquired some practical knowledge of meditation, proffered this explanation:

> [Meditative absorption] is a deepened and creative *dharana*, in which the inner object is illumined mentally. The strict concentration on one object of consciousness is now supplemented with a searching-pensive contemplation of its actual nature. The object is, so to speak, placed before the contemplative consciousness in all its aspects and is apperceived as a whole. Its

various characteristics are examined until its very essence is understood and becomes transparent. . . . This is accompanied by a certain emotive disposition. Although the reasoning faculty functions acutely and clearly, it would be wrong to understand *dhyana* merely as a logical-rational process: The contemplator must penetrate his object with all his heart, because after all he is concerned about a spiritual experience that is to lead him to the sphere of ontic participation and the liberation from all constricting and binding hindrances.[1]

These observations are complemented by the following consideration in Mircea Eliade's classic work on Yoga:

. . . this act must be conceived neither under the species of the poetic imagination, nor under that of an intuition of the Bergsonian type. What sharply distinguishes yogic meditation from these two irrational "flights" is its coherence, the state of lucidity that accompanies and continually orients it.[2]

Meditation, then, is a lucid inner state in which the flow of attention and energy revolves around a single content of consciousness, or what is commonly called an "idea." However, meditation is more than a technique or activity. It is, above all, a state of being or what the Japanese Buddhists call "just sitting"—an inner disposition that eludes precise definition. Meditation imitates the tranquil state of the Self. It is an approximation of that which is ultimately real.

This has been poignantly expressed by psychologist Claudio Naranjo when he wrote that meditation "is concerned with the development of a *presence*, a modality of being."[3] He went on as follows:

This presence or mode transforms whatever it touches. If its medium is movement, it will turn into dance; if stillness, into living sculpture; if thinking, into the higher reaches of intuition; if sensing, into a merging with the miracle of being; if feeling, into love; if singing, into sacred utterance; if speaking, into prayer or poetry; if doing the things of ordinary life, into a ritual in the name of God or a celebration of existence.[4]

In Classical Yoga, however, the purpose of meditative absorption is not dance, song, or poetry but the radical stoppage of the
fluctuations (*vritti*) of consciousness. This entails the elimination of
all cognitive, conative, and emotive activity. Patanjali distinguished five such fluctuations or "whirls": (1) knowledge arising
from perception, inference, or testimony; (2) erroneous knowledge; (3) conceptualization or phantasy; (4) sleep, and (5)
memory.[5] This grouping is by no means arbitrary but takes into
account the "distance" of the various fluctuations from the external world, with knowledge as the outermost and memory as the
most internal function.

The first two "whirls" are eliminated through sensory inhibition. Conceptualization is still present at the outset of meditation,
but gradually diminishes as the process of unification proceeds.
Undoubtedly the greatest obstacle for meditators is sleep, which
can only be overcome through unrelenting vigilance. After that,
spiritual practitioners only have to confront and inhibit the powerful human memory, which is the source of all the thoughts, emotions, and mental images occurring particularly at the beginning of
meditation.

In the last analysis, memory refers to the depth-consciousness,
or subconscious, in which all experience is stored in the form of the
so-called "activators" (samskara). In meditation the external or
"coarse" aspect of memory is blocked out.[6] Its inner or "subtle"
aspect, consisting of the samskara traces, is fully overcome only in
the highest form of spiritual realization, which is the supraconscious ecstasy called *asamprajnata-samadhi*.

The recognition that the fluctuations of consciousness do not
make up the whole dynamics of consciousness but are to be inhib-
ited already at the stage of meditation is crucial to a proper understanding of Classical Yoga and Yoga in general. Thus, the restriction aimed at in Yoga appears as a three-level process.

During the first or meditation phase of internalization the fluctuations are eliminated. During the second phase, consisting of
object-conscious ecstasy, the ideas (pratyaya) present in the ecstatic state are obliterated. During the last phase, in the condition
of supraconscious ecstasy, the karmic "seeds" in the subconscious-
ness are "sterilized." This can be tabulated as follows:

1. *vritti-nirodha* or restriction of the mental fluctuations;

2. *pratyaya-nirodha* or restriction of the ideas arising in the ecstatic state;

3. *samskara-nirodha* or restriction of the subliminal "activators."

In other words, restriction takes place on a progressively deeper (or higher) level. The periods of restriction on these three levels are naturally of varying duration, and in the beginning they tend to be extremely brief. Thus, in its initial stages, the state of meditative absorption can still be quite easily disrupted by a sudden shrill sound, a hard push, or even a strong upsetting mental sensation or image. However, with practice, both the intensity and duration of meditation increase, and the adept finds no difficulty in remaining in that condition of inwardness for many hours.

MEDITATION WITH AND WITHOUT OBJECT

Even though the actual mechanism of internalization is the same in all cases, the results and manifestations of meditation vary according to the nature of the object chosen, as well as according to individual psychological factors. Since Patanjali gave yogins a free hand in the choice of their object of concentration, and the range of possible objects is enormous, it is difficult to come up with a satisfactory classification of the meditation experiences of his followers.[7]

However, in principle, two types of meditative absorption can be distinguished, depending on whether or not a specific object is in fact employed. Object-centered meditation selects a suitable prop from the countless forms of the manifest universe, be it a mountain, a favorite saint, a higher entity such as a deity, a benign thought, one of the psychosomatic centers of the body, or a bodily function, such as the breath. The last-mentioned possibility plays a prominent role in modern Theravada Buddhism.

This angle of yogic absorption is brought out in the following report by W.L. King, who was initiated into *vipassana* meditation:

. . . To achieve this kind of meditation, we were instructed to begin with the breath-lip awareness and, when attention was fully gained there, to shift the focus to the fontanelle, which, as the coming-together point of the skull bones on the top of the head, is the "most sensitive point" in the human body. As a result of successful concentration here one begins to feel pricklings, stingings, itchings, or burnings. By widening his attention he is to "push" or "widen" this tingling area over the crown, then down the sides of the head, and finally down through the whole body. The goal is to gain such a body-awareness that a person can focus his attention on any one point in the body in such a way that separate physical sensation springs up there at will—evidenced by burning or prickling. As he grows in power to do this, he tries more and more to center his body-awareness in the heart-chest region, which is the core of man's psychophysical being, according to Buddhism, and the last refuge of those impurities he is now seeking to "destroy."[8]

There is also an objectless meditation, and this type is the favored technique of certain Tantric schools. It is described in a Tibetan text, which was edited by the British scholar and practitioner W.Y. Evans-Wentz. This work describes the approach of the *mahamudra* ("great seal") thus:

Think not of the past. Think not of the future. Think not that thou art actually engaged in meditation. Regard not the Void as being Nothingness.

At this stage do not attempt to analyse any of the impressions felt by the five senses, saying, "It is; it is not." But at least for a little while observe unbroken meditation, keeping the body as calm as that of a sleeping babe, and the mind in its natural state [i.e., free of all thought processes].[9]

The Vedantic equivalent to this Buddhist practice can be encountered in the practice of "self-inquiry, as formulated by the modern Indian sage Ramana Maharshi of Tiruvannamalai. He thought that object-centered meditation was "like a thief turning policeman to catch the thief that is himself."[10] By contrast, as Ramana saw it, self-inquiry goes straight to the core, which is the Self itself.

Self-inquiry, in the form of the probing question "Who am I?", proceeds by means of the mind but does not confuse the mind with Reality. Self-inquiry tries to ferret out the origin of the ego and mind, rather than be misled by them. Ultimately, the presumed "I" that seemingly undertakes the process of self-inquiry is transcended when the Self shines forth in its native radiance.

More conventionally, Vedanta teachers recommend objectless meditation in the form of the assertion "I am the Absolute" (*aham brahma asmi*). It is their belief that this strong conviction, combined with the renunciation of all worldly things, has the power to peel away the layers of false identification from which the unenlightened individual suffers. When pursued with sufficient rigor, this practice reveals the transcendental "I" beyond the ego. That ultimate, irreducible identity is the Self (atman).

MEDITATION AS VISUALIZATION

The objectless approach to meditation sharply contrasts with the extremely complex visualization practices generally adopted in Tantrism and Hatha-Yoga. These traditions make a distinction between "coarse meditation," "luminous meditation," and "subtle meditation." These three types are explained in the *Gheranda-Samhita* (VI.1) thus:

"Coarse" is said [to mean] "consisting of shape"; "luminous" is "consisting of light"; "subtle" is "consisting of the seed-point (*bindu*)," [which is] the Absolute, the *kundalini*, the supreme Goddess.

This explanation is followed by a model case of each type of meditative absorption. The coarse form is described in this way:

Let [the yogin] imagine that there is a great sea of nectar in his own heart; that in the middle of that [sea] there is an island of precious stones, the sand of which is pulverized gems; that on all sides of it are *nipa* trees laden with sweet flowers; that next to these trees, like a rampart, there is a row of flowering trees such as *malati, mallika*, nutmeg, *kesara, campaka*, coral, and *padma*, and that the fragrance of these flowers is spreading all round. In the middle of the grove let the yogin imagine the

beautiful *kalpa* tree with four branches representing the four
Vedas, and that it is laden with flowers and fruits. Beetles are
humming there and cuckoos are calling. Beneath that [tree] let
the yogin imagine a great platform of precious gems. Let the
yogin [further] imagine that in its middle there is a beautiful
throne inlaid with jewels. On that [throne] let the yogin imagine his particular deity, as taught by the teacher [who will instruct him as to] the appropriate form, adornment and vehicle
of that deity. Such a form constantly meditated upon—know
this to be coarse meditation.[11]

The nature of luminous meditation can be gathered from the
following instruction:

In the root center (*muladhara*), the *kundalini* rests in the shape of
a serpent. There is the individual consciousness resembling
the light of a lamp. [Concentrating on it], one should contemplate the luminous Absolute. [This is] luminous meditation,
[which is] more excellent than the previous [practice of coarse
meditation].[12]

An alternative exercise is the absorption into the light of the
sixth psychoenergetic center (*ajna-cakra*) by fixing the gaze between the eyebrows. Absorption by means of light phenomena is
the salient feature of *taraka-yoga*, the "Yoga of the Deliverer." This
approach is expounded in the *Advaya-Taraka-Upanishad* and the
Mandala-Brahmana-Upanishad, which are creations of the medieval
period.

This little known but at one time apparently widely practiced
form of Yoga is the counterpart of *nada-yoga* in which mainly audi-
tory phenomena are employed to achieve psychomental unification.

The subtle meditation, which is deemed a hundred thousand
times more valuable than its "luminous" equivalent, is apparently
identical with the celebrated practice of *shambhavi-mudra*, in which
the consciousness is focused in the heart center while the eyes are
kept open.[13]

The place given to meditative absorption in Yoga is comparable to intensive mental prayer in the spiritual practice of Christianity. This act is understood as the uplifting of one's soul by way of surrendered concentration.

Indeed, without disciplined turning inward of the mind, the ultimate goal of perfect self-transcendence and Self-realization remains an abstract concept. Hence the *Garuda-Purana* (222.10) declares:

> Meditation is the highest virtue. Meditation is the highest austerity. Meditation is the highest purity. Therefore be fond of meditation.

Echoing the same sentiment, Shankara said about meditation that it is a thousand times more valuable than mere intellectual reflection.[14] Its great value lies in that it leads to one's merger with the contemplated object. No mere intellectual knowledge can accomplish this. Meditation is the steep path to the mountain peak of enlightenment, or liberation.

Gautama the Buddha practiced terrifying self-mortification for many years before it dawned on him that there was a much simpler way: to still body and mind, and allow focused attention to work the great miracle of transcendence. For a single night he sat under the fig tree, fighting with his own inner demons and penetrating the levels of cosmic existence until he had reached his destination. When he rose from his seat at dawn, he was as radiant as the rising sun. He had awakened from the dream of life.

NOTES

1. J.W. Hauer, *Der Yoga: Ein indischer Weg zum Selbst* (Stuttgart: Kohlhammer Verlag, 1958), p. 322.

2. M. Eliade, *Yoga: Immortality and Freedom* (Princeton, NJ: Princeton University Press, 1970), p. 73.

3. C. Naranjo in C. Naranjo and R.E. Ornstein, *On the Psychology of Meditation* (London: Allen & Unwin, 1971), p. 8.

4. *Ibid.*, p. 8.

5. See *Yoga-Sutra* I.5–11.

6. See *Yoga-Sutra* II.11.

7. See *Yoga-Sutra* I.39.

8. W.L. King, *A Thousand Lives Away* (Oxford: Cassirer, 1964), pp. 228–229.

9. W.Y. Evans-Wentz, ed., *Tibetan Yoga and Secret Doctrines* (London/Oxford: Oxford University Press, 1967), p. 119. The quotation is from the *Epitome of the Great Symbol* (I.13–14).

10. A. Osborne, ed., *The Collected Works of Ramana Maharshi* (New York: Weiser, 1970), p. 112.

11. *Gheranda-Samhita* VI.2–8.

12. *Gheranda-Samhita* VI.16.

13. See *Gheranda-Samhita* VI.21.

14. See *Viveka-Cudamani*, verse 364.

CHAPTER 20

THE ECSTATIC CONSCIOUSNESS: GOING BEYOND SUBJECT AND OBJECT

ECSTASY AS SPONTANEOUS BREAKTHROUGH

As we have seen, the mythic orientation to spirituality is world- and ego-negating. Its most important accomplishment is the unitive experience in which subject and object are perfectly merged. In most Indian traditions this state is known as *samadhi*, which can be rendered as "ecstasy."[1] In his well-known commentary on the *Yoga-Sutra* (I.1), Vyasa even defines Yoga as samadhi.[2] In other words, Yoga is what we would call a mystical tradition, which revolves around the attainment of self-transcendence through the ecstatic condition.

This extraordinary modality of consciousness ensues with the perfect pacification of the "whirls" of consciousness during the state of meditative absorption. However, it would be quite wrong to conceive of the ecstatic breakthrough as a necessary causal consequence of the meditative emptying of the mind. The ecstatic realization pertains to an ontic level that is completely distinct from that of either meditation or ordinary consciousness. The transition from the state of absorption to ecstasy is an abrupt and sudden break, leading to a new mode of being.

That break, or rupture, is effected by a force that seemingly comes from "within" or "above." The theistic schools have interpreted this happening as an influx of divine grace (prasada). But even in nontheistic schools, this event is considered to be unpredictable.

This significant fact, namely that ecstasy cannot be brought about by sheer willpower, appears to be confirmed by the drug experiments of recent years. Hallucinogenic compounds such as LSD 25 or mescaline are unable to predictably produce ecstatic states of consciousness. They do affect our nervous system and thereby drastically change the way in which we perceive the world, at least until their chemical effect on the body has worn off. However, their operation is largely restricted to the level of sensory activity.

For instance, synaesthetic experiences, in which forms, colors, and sounds are all crosswired, are fascinating and may give one a new understanding of the world; they are not, however, mystical experiences. Even the sense of oneness with one's environment, which has been reported by some drug takers, is only the merest intimation of the ecstatic state.

In cases where genuine mystical experiences have occurred, the drug simply acted as a catalyst. We may safely assume that prolonged meditation, breathing, listening to music, or making love might have proved a similarly potent trigger.

At any rate, the "slot-meter" view that drugs can induce the highest mystical experiences is a dangerous misrepresentation. As numerous studies have borne out, psychedelic drugs can bring into consciousness only what is in one form or another already preexistent in it. Hence researchers have emphasized the importance of both setting and set, the latter term referring to the psychological state of the individual.

In his book *Drugs of Hallucination*, Sidney Cohen addresses this matter squarely when he writes:

> It is tempting to say that one gets from the LSD encounter what one deserves, but this is not so. Seven centuries ago St. Thomas Aquinas said it more accurately: "Quid quid recipiteur secundum modum recipientis recipiteur": We get, not what we deserve, but what we are. A pill does not construct character, educate the emotions or improve intelligence. It is not a spiritual labour-saving device, salvation, instant wisdom, or a short cut to maturity.[3]

Similarly, the ecstatic consciousness visits those who sufficiently resonate with the unitive state of being. Ascetics may spend a lifetime trying to procure it and yet not once enjoy its delight and simplicity. Or again, a person who has had no formal preparation in spiritual matters may, out of the blue, be overcome by the ecstatic condition. The occurrence of the ecstatic state is embedded in a great mystery.

Nevertheless, ecstasy is not a random event either. There are laws or regularities at work, but these fall outside the orbit of ordinary understanding. Moreover, there is one identifiable precondition to ecstasy. That is the gesture of self-surrender. A person who is inclined to yield his or her hold on the body-mind, or ego-personality, creates a favorable climate for the ecstatic breakthrough.

In 1964, John Blofeld, an expert on and practitioner of Tibetan Buddhism, allowed himself to be talked into experimenting with mescaline.[4] About an hour after taking the first half of a dose of the drug, he began to experience a process that threatened to disintegrate his sense of self. He was struggling against it, all the while feeling very tense. This gave way to lethargy. Upon taking the second half of the dose, Blofeld found himself back in an overwhelming sensation of self-fragmentation. He became paranoid about his condition, fearing that he had succumbed to madness.

Three hours into the experience, Blofeld retired to his bedroom, shutting himself away from everyone "like a sick animal." His inner tension had grown so strong that his only desire was to rid himself of it, whether it be by fleeing into madness or embracing death. With this resolution, he suddenly found himself able to let go completely. He surrendered to the situation and, promptly, found himself on the other side of all the inner turmoil and pain. From what he described as a state of hell, he entered into indescribable ecstasy.

Blofeld was unable to explain why the drug was able to elicit an experience that had eluded him despite his many years of spiritual discipline. He failed to see that it may well have been his long Buddhist training that empowered him to surrender the ego at the critical moment.

UNDERSTANDING THE STATE OF ECSTATIC UNDIVIDEDNESS

The nature of ecstasy can be communicated only with great difficulty, because this experience explodes the categories of ordinary logic. In the final analysis, we can only comprehend the ecstatic state through personal realization. As Zen master and scholar D.T. Suzuki noted:

It is an experience which even a mountain of explanations

and proofs cannot bring home to others, except if they themselves have had this experience.[5]

Many centuries ago, Vyasa expressed the same idea when he remarked, "Yoga can be understood [only] through Yoga."[6] Agreeing with this sentiment, Mircea Eliade interjected this warning:

> Denial of the reality of the yogic experience, or criticism of certain of its aspects, is inadmissible from a man who has no direct knowledge of its practice, for yogic states go beyond the condition that circumscribes us when we criticize them.[7]

This proviso is chiefly directed to psychologists, whose academic training makes them inclined to deny *a priori* the authenticity of the ecstatic experience and to see in it merely a hypnotic or cataleptic state, schizophrenia, or a similar abnormal mental condition. From a purely physiological viewpoint, it is correct to maintain that when the lower forms of yogic ecstasy ensue, a state similar to catalepsy occurs. However, this is not the whole truth. The external rigidity fails to portray the simultaneous richness of the internal experience.

The favorite scientific explanation that this state is merely a relapse into unconsciousness not only contradicts all the statements in the spiritual literature but also ignores the testimony of the mystics of all ages. For, without exception, they speak of an extreme lucidity of consciousness during ecstasy. Thus, the Yoga masters were careful to distinguish between genuine ecstasy and pseudo-ecstatic states, which may rightly be equated with relapses into unconsciousness, called *jadya* in Sanskrit.

In this connection mention must be made of the well-known feat, demonstrated by some yogins or fakirs, of being buried for several hours or even days in an apparently airtight box. They induce a psychosomatic state very similar to hibernation, which goes by the name of *jada-samadhi*, meaning "insentient ecstasy." However, this is merely a psychological curiosity; it has no intrinsic spiritual value. Genuine ecstasy, as Ramana Maharshi put it, is always "waking sleep" (*jagrat-sushupti*), without any trace of obscuration or diminished awareness.

In light of the numerous firsthand accounts of this experience that are available today, the psychological interpretation proffered many years ago by C.G. Jung, which continues to be evoked in some quarters, likewise proves inadequate. He said:

> One hopes to dominate the unconscious, but the past masters of this art of domination—the yogis—wind up with samadhi, an ecstatic condition that seems to be equivalent to an unconscious state. The fact that they call our unconscious the universal consciousness, does not change things in the least: in their case the unconscious has devoured the ego-consciousness. They do not realize that exclusiveness, selection, and discrimination are the root and essence of all that can claim the name of consciousness.[8]

Jung further argued that the "universal consciousness" of Eastern traditions cannot be anything but the psychologist's "unconscious." He did not deny that the methods of Buddhism and Yoga help one achieve an expansion of consciousness, but, for him, an infinitely extended consciousness must necessarily be diffuse and dim and hence undesirable. He summarized his thoughts by saying, "This is all very well, but scarcely to be recommended anywhere north of the Tropic of Cancer."

In his consideration of this important matter, Jung chose logic and opinion over personal experimentation. Not surprisingly, his dismissal of samadhi as "vast but dim" has found little sympathy in Eastern quarters. For instance, in his book *Hindu Psychology*, Swami Akhilananda commented on Jung's observation as follows:

> Any man who has had these realizations will laugh at such conclusions. Patanjali, Swami Vivekananda, and Swami Brahmananda give just the opposite point of view. They make it clear that *samadhi*, or the superconscious state, is vivid and definite. It is indeed true that in certain superconscious states . . . the perceiver, perceived, and knowledge . . . are wholly identified. All the differences vanish in the integral unity. This happens because all the manifestations merge at that time in one Absolute Existence without differentiation of any kind. So the superconscious is not unconscious; it is full of awareness; nay, it is Consciousness Itself.[9]

Swami Akhilananda went on to characterize Jung's views on the matter as superficial. He remarked that before the super-conscious state can be reached, one must have controlled, inte-grated, and "wholly emptied" the contents of the unconscious. While it is doubtful that the unconscious can ever be emptied, the learned swami is right in insisting that the ecstatic state must not be confused with the unconscious.

Jung's position was also criticized by some Western psycholo-gists with a practical knowledge of Eastern traditions. Thus, the Australian psychotherapist Hans Jacobs, a former pupil of Jung, felt urged to make the following strong comments:

> Jung's whole attitude here is emotionally conditioned and not unprejudiced. It may be that he is so impressed by his own discoveries that he permits nothing else to intrude upon him. It is also possible that he feels some omission in his own life.[10]

That Jung's own system is not as logically sound as he would have us believe is evident from his later admission that the uncon-scious possesses a relative consciousness after all. His dualistic ap-proach to the psyche proved ill-equipped for elucidating the ec-static state. If anything, it tended to obscure it.

Similarly untenable and unconstructive is the once-fashion-able hypnosis theory. The attempt of some scholars to explain ec-stasy as a hypnotic condition is as one-sided as it is absurd, in view of the statements to the contrary made by those who have person-ally experienced it. The Yoga scriptures quite clearly distinguish between ecstatic and hypnotic states.[11]

The German Yoga researcher J.W. Hauer first protested against this irresponsible hypothesis, although he made the mistake of characterizing the hypnotic state as one of unconsciousness.[12] As his countryman Dietrich Langen, a professor of psychiatry, pointed out, the hypnotic state involves a certain "twilight" or "standby" consciousness, so that one can even speak of the hyp-notic state as one of partial wakefulness.[13]

However, to apply the same term to the ecstatic state, as Langen has done, is more than misleading. He seems to have sensed this because he freely admits that ecstasy is accompanied by a "luminous supra-wakefulness." He appears to vacillate between the academic hypnosis theory and the yogic claim for the complete otherness of ecstasy, and his description of samadhi as a "hypnoid sub-wakeful state" which contains a "supra-wakeful consciousness center" contributes nothing to the solution of this problem.

Finally, the equation of ecstasy with schizophrenic or psychotic states of mind deserves no special refutation. The words of the famous Tantric teacher Saraha, who lived in the eighth century A.D., will suffice to correct this erroneous notion:

Do not think the mind is sick when there is ecstasy—for this is only what appears to the ordinary people.[14]

DEFINING THE ELUSIVE STATE

After these preliminary observations, it will be possible to give the texts themselves a hearing. The classic definition of the nature of the ecstatic state is to be found in Patanjali's *Yoga-Sutra* (III.3):

[When] this [object of meditation] shines forth as the sole reality [and consciousness is] as it were devoid of its essence— [that is] ecstasy.

The Sanskrit commentators have interpreted this aphorism slightly differently. They take the first word, *tad* ("this"), to refer not to the object of consciousness but to meditation itself, which makes little sense. For how could meditative absorption shine forth as the sole reality? Also, the phrase *sva-rupa-shunyam-iva* ("as it were devoid of [its] essence") is erroneously linked to meditation instead of consciousness.

While Vyasa, the earliest commentator whose work has survived, deals with this important aphorism only very cursorily, Vacaspati Mishra quotes an interesting passage from the *Vishnu-Purana* (VI.7.90):

The grasping of the essence of this [supreme God Vishnu] without [any] conceptualization, [as it is] achieved with the mind in [the state of] meditation—that is called ecstasy.[15]

And in his fifteenth-century *Panca-Dashi* (I.55), Vidyaranya states:

By gradually giving up [the distinction between] meditator and meditation, the sphere of the object alone [shines forth in consciousness], and consciousness resembles a lamp in a windless [place]—[that] is designated as ecstasy.

The *Laghu-Yoga-Vasishtha* (III.118), again, has the following definition:

That state [of consciousness], in which all volition has ceased completely [and which is] like the interior of a stone [but at the same time] free from unconsciousness and sleep—[that] is called the state of the essence [of consciousness].

Similar statements can be found in many Hindu scriptures that deal with the higher stages of the spiritual path, and all the definitions of samadhi are essentially the same. They emphasize the ecstatic merging with the object, which looms large in consciousness, whatever the object of contemplation may be.

In the *Yoga-Sutra*, the lower forms of ecstasy—those that are connected with an object other than the transcendental Subject—also bear the technical name *samapatti*. This word means "falling together" or "coincidence," which describes the central happening in ecstasy very well. For the ecstatic consciousness is characterized by the object of contemplation filling out the entire space of awareness. In ecstasy, there is no longer any experience of externality.

Consciousness is said to become like a crystal that reflects the color of the base on which its rests.[16] The focal point of the ecstatic consciousness can be either the transcendental Subject or Self, or any of the multitude of objects in the realm of cosmic existence, including the process of apperception itself.[17]

According to King Bhoja, who defined ecstasy as a "special contemplation," the contents of ecstatic consciousness can be either the Lord (ishvara), or the Self, or else Nature.[18] This tripartition corresponds to the differentiation of the mystical experience, as established by the British historian of religion R.C. Zaehner:

1. the apperception of God, or the beatific vision;
2. the identification with the Self;
3. the identification with the non-Self.[19]

To recapitulate: At the moment of extreme inner immobility, that is, with the disengagement of the mental machinery in meditation, the necessary vacuum is created for the ecstatic consciousness to break through. Then the subject-object barrier peculiar to the empirical consciousness is removed, and the object of absorption is suddenly no longer merely ideated, but becomes a living reality with which consciousness coincides to the extent that the experiencing subject, the experienced object, and the process of experience merge into a single field.

We become, in consciousness, the bird we contemplate; we become the tree in which the sap circulates and which stretches its ramified crown toward the invigorating sun; we become the solar disk whose vivifying energies pour over the planets of our galaxy; we become the universe in its grand immensity and pulsating fullness. We may even become one with the tranquil center in the depths of our own being, or unite with the all-comprising wholeness of the supreme Being. On whatever level such ontic identification takes place, it always presupposes the abolition of the ordinary space-time continuum and the experience of the eternal Now.

THE LADDER OF ECSTATIC UNIFICATION

From this it can be seen that the ecstatic state is by no means the uniform phenomenon it has generally been supposed to be. On the contrary, it is an extraordinary multiform experience. The Yoga texts distinguish between two essentially distinct types of ecstasy: ontic identification connected with object consciousness (*samprajnata-samadhi*) and ontic identification with the subjective core unaccompanied by object consciousness (*asamprajnata-samadhi*).

In Vedanta, the synonyms *savikalpa-samadhi* and *nirvikalpa-samadhi* are used respectively. The former type of ecstasy still contains a variety of conscious contents, while in the second and higher type, consciousness is transmuted into, or superseded by, transcendental Awareness.

Patanjali has bequeathed to us an interesting phenomenological scheme, which is of vital importance in all schools of Yoga operating within the framework of Samkhya ontology rather than the idealist metaphysics of Vedanta. According to the information

given in the *Yoga-Sutra*, the various grades of ecstatic realization
may be tabulated as follows:

A. Ecstasy with an objective prop (*samprajnata-samadhi*), or
   conscious ecstasy:

    1. *vitarka-samadhi*, or ontic identification with the external
   or "coarse" (*sthula*) aspect of the object of contemplation,
   which is connected with certain awarenesses (*pratyaya*), as
   explained on the following pages;

    2. *nirvitarka-samadhi*, or ontic identification with the exter-
   nal or coarse aspect of the object of contemplation, which is
   without arising awarenesses;

    3. *vicara-samadhi*, or ontic identification with the inner or
   "subtle" (*sukshma*) aspect of the object of contemplation,
   which is connected with awarenesses;

    4. *nirvicara-samadhi*, or ontic identification with the inner or
   subtle aspect of the object of contemplation, which is without any arising awarenesses.

B. Ecstasy without objective prop (*asamprajnata-samadhi*), or
   supraconscious ecstasy:

    This ecstatic state has no subdivisions, as it does not have
   different possible objects of contemplation.

It is virtually impossible to express the full meaning of the Sanskrit terms *samprajnata* and *asamprajnata* by single English words.
The usual rendering of *prajna* as "cognition" must be used with
caution, because in the samadhi state there is, strictly speaking, no
experience of an object. The subject *becomes* the object, or the object
fills out the subject.

The term prajna literally means "knowing beyond," that is,
transcendental realization based on the coincidence of subject and
object. Hence samprajnata-samadhi, or conscious ecstasy, may be
described as that ecstatic experience in which transcendental cognitive activity occurs. This activity is not to be confused with the
familiar thought-processes, because these must have been thoroughly controlled through concentration and meditation before

the switch from the empirical to the ecstatic consciousness can occur.

What exactly, then, are these "arising awarenesses," the recurring noetic acts in ecstasy? First of all, they are not identical with the ordinary thought-associations that meander on automatically like viscous liquid. Rather, they represent something intrinsically novel. They have a palpable immediacy that distinguishes them from the usual vague ramblings of the mind confronting an object. They are pure thought, instant recognitions, or certainties of understanding.

They are suprawakeful knowing, a form of thinking that is not identical with the sense-based semiconscious activity of the ordinary mind. They are spontaneous and transparent flashes of awareness and understanding, born of the unmediated experience of the object of contemplation.

These supercognitions fall into two major categories, according to the ontic level on which the object is experienced in ecstasy, namely *vitarka* ("cogitation") and *vicara* ("reflection"). In vitarka-samadhi, the external or coarse aspect of the object is ecstatically apprehended. This unmediated apprehension (*sakshatkara*) is not confined to the present structure of the object of contemplation. As Vijnana Bhikshu explained in his *Yoga-Sara-Samgraha* (chapter I), it extends over the object's past and future form. Upon cessation of all noetic activity in this ecstatic state, nirvitarka-samadhi ensues.

In vicara-samadhi, the practitioner's consciousness penetrates into the very essence of the object thus disclosing its deeper ontic stratum. What this means can only be understood within the framework of the ontology of Yoga and Samkhya: Cosmic reality, called prakriti, is not only that which can be perceived with the senses; it also includes an inner or subtle dimension that is hierarchically stratified.

This invisible realm extends from Nature's pure matrix of potentiality to the ontic plane of the logos or higher mind (buddhi) and, further still, to the psychic realities of the "I-maker" (*ahamkara* or *asmita*), the sense-bound lower mind (*manas*), the senses (*indriya*), and the energetic forces (*tanmatra*) underlying the coarse elements (*bhuta*) that compose the visible universe. This ancient model seeks to explain the evolution from the One to the Many, and in this form was originally the result of meditative and ecstatic introspection.

In vicara-samadhi, the interiority of the object of contemplation is exposed, and when in this state all noetic activity also comes to a standstill, the practitioner enters nirvicara-samadhi. At the peak of this ecstatic consciousness occurs what the *Yoga-Sutra* (I.47) describes as the "autumnal lucidity."[20] At this point the supercognition is said to become "truth-bearing" (*ritam-bhara*).[21]

The culmination of conscious ecstasy, which is connected with an objective prop, is reached when the personality core (sattva) shines forth unblurred, with a degree of translucency comparable to that of the Self. Here is the threshold that leads to the nonobjective, supraconscious ecstasy revealing the Self, or Spirit, itself.

The avenue for rediscovering the innate freedom of the transcendental Self, the eternal Witness, is the elimination of all the traces that our life experiences have left behind in the deeps of consciousness. This is accomplished in asamprajnata-samadhi, or supraconscious ecstasy. This elusive state progressively burns out all subliminal residua responsible for the formation of consciousness and thus of duality and alienation from the Self.

In this ecstatic state takes place the total remolding of the human being into the transcendental Being-Awareness. This radical self-transcending process finds its conclusion in the so-called "seedless ecstasy" (*nirbija-samadhi*), in which the return into the semiconsciousness of the ordinary waking state is rendered impossible and the yogin becomes emancipated.

The ultimate ecstasy is also referred to as *dharma-megha-samadhi*, or "ecstasy of the cloud of dharma." It is not clear in what sense the word *dharma* is used in this context. The classical exegetes have interpreted it as "virtue," and this explanation seems to have satisfied most scholars. However, in view of the fact that the liberated being is said to have transcended good and evil, this interpretation does not ring quite true. I have therefore elsewhere suggested that dharma here refers to the primary constituents (guna) of the world ground.[22]

If this interpretation is correct, we can then understand dharma-megha-samadhi as that very last moment at the culmination of the process of ecstatic involution in which the yogin is separated from transcendental Awareness merely by a thin veil, as it were, namely, the "cloud" of the primary constituents which are in the process of resolving back into the world ground.

The ecstatic states transport the adept to increasingly deeper (or "higher") dimensions of the vast organism of Nature. They proceed from the realm of countless particulars to the universal, that is, the ultimately Real, which is the Self. This process of involution takes place in distinct stages, which can be understood in terms of levels of achievement of varying degrees of difficulty. Vacaspati Mishra, in his *Tattva-Vaisharadi* (I.17), compares the yogin practicing ecstasy to an archer who shoots at increasingly smaller and more distant targets. However, such scales of ecstatic involution are intended to serve as general map only, and are seldom strictly adhered to in practice.

In addition, it is commonly assumed that by the grace of God or through the blessings of the teacher, aspirants are enabled to skip one or more stages.[23] Moreover, in the lower levels of ecstasy, there are no fixed boundaries between one state and another, and this permits the accomplished adept to move consciously up and down the ecstatic scale.

To summarize the above consideration, we can say that the polymorphous ecstatic realization connected with object consciousness shows three constants: suprawakefulness, peace, and ontic identification. These ingredients are all germinally present already in the state of meditative absorption. As meditation deepens, the wall between contemplator and contemplated object increasingly crumbles.

In the ultimate ecstatic condition, which is devoid of object consciousness, even these three characteristics are transcended. What remains is pure Self-Awareness, the immovable Witness of all phenomena.

NOTES

1. Mircea Eliade preferred the term "enstasy," and in my more scholarly works I have adopted this coinage, because it is somewhat more appropriate. Samadhi is not about being beside oneself, which is the common

connotation of "ecstasy." Rather, it is an abiding in one's center. This aspect is better conveyed by the Greek term *enstasis*, which literally means "standing in (oneself)."

2. See *Yoga-Bhashya* I.1.

3. See S. Cohen, *Drugs of Hallucination: The Uses and Misuses of Lysergic Acid Diethylamide* (London: Paladin, 1965), p. 240.

4. J. Blofeld, "Consciousness, Energy, Bliss," in R. Metzner, ed., *The Ecstatic Adventure* (New York: Macmillan, 1968), pp. 124-133.

5. D.T. Suzuki, *Die grosse Befreiung* (Zurich/Stuttgart, 1958), p. 127.

6. *Yoga-Bhashya* III.6.

7. M. Eliade, *Yoga: Immortality and Freedom* (Princeton, NJ: Princeton University Press, 1970), p. 39.

8. C.G. Jung, *The Integration of the Personality* (London: Kegan Paul, 1963), p. 26.

9. Swami Akhilananda, *Hindu Psychology: Its Meaning for the West* (London: Routledge & Sons, 1947), p. 167.

10. H. Jacobs, *Western Therapy and Hindu Sadhana: A Contribution to Comparative Studies in Psychology and Metaphysics* (London: Allen & Unwin, 1961), p. 164.

11. See the pertinent remarks in M. Eliade, *Yoga: Immortality and Freedom*, pp. 76–79.

12. See J.W. Hauer, *Der Yoga: Ein indischer Weg zum Selbst* (Stuttgart: Kohlhammer, 1958).

13. D. Langen, *Archaische Ekstase und Asiatische Meditation* (Stuttgart: Hippokrates-Verlag, 1963).

14. *Doha-Kosha*, chapter III (Hindi edition by R. Samkrtyayana), quoted in A. Bharati, *The Tantric Tradition* (London: Rider, 1970), p. 290.

15. Quoted in the *Tattva-Vaisharadi* III.3.

16. See *Yoga-Sutra* I.41.

17. *Yoga-Sutra* III.47.

18. See *Raja-Martanda* I.17.

19. See R.C. Zaehner, *Mysticism: Sacred and Profane* (Oxford: Oxford University Press, 1957), p. 22. Cf. N. Smart's stimulating criticism of Zaehner's arguments in *The Yogi and the Devotee: The Interplay between the Upanishads and Catholic Theology* (London: Allen & Unwin, 1968), pp. 66ff.

20. The Sanskrit term is *vaisharadya*, which is derived from "autumn" (*sharad*), the clearest season in Northern India.

21. See *Yoga-Sutra* I.48.

22. See G. Feuerstein, *The Philosophy of Classical Yoga* (Manchester: Manchester University Press, 1980), pp. 98–101. This interpretation of *dharma-megha-samadhi* is of course purely conjectural and stands in need of verification. It could also be that the author of the *Yoga-Sutra* employed this expression, which has a distinct Buddhist flavor, in exactly the sense it is given for example in the *Sad-Dharma-Pundarika-Sutra* (chapter V).

23. See *Yoga-Sara-Samgraha*, chapter II.

CHAPTER 21

ALLUREMENT THROUGH MAGICAL POWERS

OBSTACLES ON THE PATH

The spiritual path to freedom may be direct but it is seldom smooth. Practitioners are apt to encounter all kinds of obstacles, which can divert them from their desired goal. We have heard about some of these hindrances in connection with the practice of concentration. As we have also seen, they can be remedied through steady adherence to the spiritual principles.

There is, however, another type of hazard on the spiritual path, which usually shows itself at a more advanced stage of practice and is therefore potentially also far more damaging to one who is heedless of it. This is the acquisition of paranormal or magical powers and the temptation they represent.

The existence of occult powers is recognized in all spiritual traditions. As Mircea Eliade noted, there is a "perfect continuity of paranormal experience from the primitive right up to the most highly evolved religions."[1] Spiritual adepts are almost universally thought to be endowed with such powers. In many traditions, however, the miraculous abilities are rejected as running counter to the spiritual work.

In Hinduism, these extraordinary abilities are known as *siddhis* ("accomplishments") or *vibhutis* ("manifestations"). They are regarded as side products of intense spiritual practice. Even though they are signs of success, they can prove a fatal trap. They are in fact a crucial test of the advanced practitioner's moral fiber and his or her commitment to self-transcendence rather than self-fulfillment, to ecstasy and freedom rather than pleasure and dependence on the world.

In those who are not firmly grounded in the moral principles of spiritual life, these miraculous powers tend to invite back all the negative and unwholesome personality traits, such as pride and hedonism, that the yogins had to renounce in order to reach their elevated position. Above all, they encourage the tendency toward extroversion, which began the karmic cycle the first place. In other words, the magical powers entice the yogins to become reinvolved with the world they once aspired to transcend.

The paranormal abilities confront the advanced practitioners with the following twofold choice. They can either assume mastery over the universe and thus fulfill the ego-personality's hunger for power and domination, or they can ignore these abilities and their own egoic promptings and continue to pursue the path of world negation and renunciation.

Folklore and mythology have spun stories of ascetics of high attainment who plummeted from their advantageous position through sheer heedlessness, folly, and the abuse of their magical faculties. There is rarely such a happy ending as in the case of the great Tibetan ascetic and poet Milarepa. While still in his youth, Milarepa was an accomplished magician, capable of conjuring up hailstorms and tempests. In this way he had caused much suffering and harm to others. Later, when he met his teacher Marpa, he was forced to undergo many years of systematic ill-treatment in order to atone for his sins. Several times, his teacher drove him to the brink of utter despair. In the end, however, Milarepa obtained the hoped for initiation, and in due course he gained enlightenment, becoming a benign and healing influence in the world.

THE SUPER-POWERS

As the whole history of Yoga bears out, the masses have always venerated and feared the yogins as powerful sorcerers. Their astonishing control over the nervous system is, from the yogic point of view, the least noteworthy achievement. Through their contemplative disciplines, they gain access to the invisible dimension, modern physics' "implicate order." From there, they appear to be able to influence the body-mind and the cosmos at large in ways that are as yet unknown to science.

These paranormal abilities are fully acknowledged by Patanjali, who mentions a considerable number of them in his *Yoga-Sutra* (chapter III). Yet, his catalogue is by no means exhaustive. The major siddhis result from the practice of ecstatic identification with a

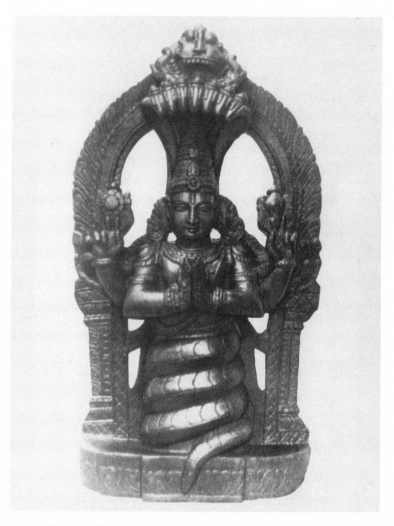

Statue of Patanjali, an incarnation of the World Serpent.
By courtesy of Sri B.K.S. Iyengar.

particular object. To mention but a few: knowledge of the past and the future, knowledge of one's former existences, knowledge of the consciousness of other beings, the ability to make oneself invisible, knowledge of what is hidden and of the inner dimension of reality, knowledge of the structure of the universe, of the stars, of the body, and so forth. At the highest level, the yogin is said to gain lordship over the entire creation.

In addition, Patanjali knows of certain magical attainments that accrue from strict observation of the rules of moral restraint and the practice of breath control. For example, by means of the steady cultivation of the virtue of nonharming, adepts are said to create around them an aura of peace that effectively neutralizes all feelings of enmity in their presence. By virtue of their nonhankering after the possessions of others, all kinds of treasures accrue to them effortlessly, and so on.

Furthermore, Patanjali states that the accomplished yogin is able to project himself into another body and travel in the "ether" (*akasha*). The latter ability probably refers to what is today known as "astral projection," for which there appears to be some experimental evidence.

The crowning magical achievement is undoubtedly the acquisition of the eight great powers (*maha-siddhi*) hinted at in the *Yoga-Sutra* (III.45). According to the *Yoga-Bhashya* (III.45), they comprise the following paranormal abilities:

1. *animan*— the ability to become as minute as an atom
2. *laghiman* — levitation
3. *mahiman* — the ability to expand infinitely
4. *prapti*— the power to reach everywhere
5. *prakamya* — freedom of will
6. *vashitva* — dominion over the entire creation
7. *ishitritva* — the power to create
8. *kama-avasayitva* — the gift of wish-fulfillment

In the *Markandeya-Purana* (XL.29–30), these occult powers are said to be indicative of one's perfect realization of the Self. The perfected adepts are widely thought to assimilate the powers of the Creator. There is, however, no agreement about whether these eight siddhis must be understood as purely subjective and

metaphorical or as actual, objective occurrences. Very revealing
in this connection is a statement attributed to Yajnavalkya, a
celebrated teacher in epic times:

> In the Vedas, the wise declare that Yoga bestows the eight
> excellences [i.e., magical powers], and they say that the eight
> excellences [belong to] the subtle [body], not to the other [i.e.,
> the physical body].[2]

That is to say, Yajnavalkya claims here that the great
paranormal abilities have nothing to do with the physical dimension. They are only true of the subtle (or astral) body, which can
shrink and expand at will. This is not the popular view, however,
which ascribes to adepts total control over the visible cosmos.

Whatever interpretation we give to these occult powers, we
must regard them as an integral element of the spiritual path. They
are not merely negative by-products, as has often been asserted,
but lawful phenomena of successful practice. They are comparable
to the ecstatic realization (samadhi), which is also only a means
and not an end in itself. Both powers and ecstasy must ultimately
be surpassed in order to reach emancipation. As the *Mahabharata*
epic (XII.196.20b) declares, "[When] ecstasy occurs in meditation,
then this [state] must also gradually be abandoned."

Ecstatic identification with the object of contemplation is a
special state of consciousness. It must not be confused with the ultimate realization of the Self. Even the highest form of ecstasy,
which in Yoga is known as asamprajnata-samadhi or "supraconscious ecstasy," is a transitional experience. Consciousness (citta)
itself must be transcended in favor of the ultimate Self-Awareness
(cit).

There is never any question that the magical powers can only
be exercised when the empirical consciousness is in full swing.
Hence they must likewise be transcended for the event of liberation to take place. However, the powers are no more obstacles
on the spiritual path than is ecstasy itself. It is, rather, the yogins'
attitude toward either that determines their further progress.

The conventional belittlement of the paranormal abilities,
especially as urged by some teachers of Advaita Vedanta, is unjus-

tified. This view is based on the mistaken assumption that the siddhis are intrinsically harmful or demonic.[3] The *Yoga-Sutra* (III.37) contains one aphorism that is regularly quoted as discrediting the paranormal powers. Yet, Patanjali would hardly have placed this aphorism in the middle of his long list of magical abilities if he had meant it to be a comprehensive denial of their usefulness.

From the context, it seems more reasonable to understand this particular aphorism as referring to the immediately preceding statement. This is also the unanimous opinion of the classical Sanskrit commentators. The two aphorisms in question run as follows.

Then occur "intuitions" [in the sensory realms of] hearing, sensing, sight, taste, and smell.—These are obstacles to ecstasy, [but] attainments in the waking [state].[4]

These intuitions (*pratibha*), or heightened sense activities, indicate that the yogin has made progress on the path of unification. They are both a blessing and a curse, because they encourage as well as tempt. Therefore, those who have acquired such abilities must not succumb to their enticement, which would merely stimulate the "whirls" of consciousness and disturb the inner peace. Thus, according to the *Yoga-Shikha-Upanishad* (I.156), the powers should always be kept carefully concealed, unless they are used for the benefit of others. Their display, in other words, would only encourage the beast of egotism to rear its head.

The acquisition of power brings with it a parallel increase in responsibility, and spiritual practitioners can only guard themselves against the temptation of misusing their newly won dominance by keeping their sight firmly fixed on the supreme Power, which is the transcendental Reality.

The power that accrues to the yogins can either catapult them out of conditioned existence into the Unconditioned, or else destroy them if they should lose sight of the supreme goal. They are as it were under a magical constraint to complete the spiritual work they have begun.

As is to be expected, the attitude of the mythic traditions of spirituality toward magical attainments is entirely negative. The

view of Advaita Vedanta has already been mentioned. The attitude
of early Buddhism is on the whole similar. In the *Digha-Nikaya*
(I.212), for instance, the Buddha is said to have made this remark:

> Because I can see the danger in the application of the magical
> powers, I reject them and despise them and am ashamed of
> them.

Everything that can divert spiritual practitioners from their intended goal must be instantly dismissed from the mind. In mythic
spirituality, this means the world in its entirety. It necessarily also
means the occult powers, which are of that world.

NOTES

1. See M. Eliade, *Myths, Dreams and Mysteries: The Encounter Between Contemporary Faiths and Archaic Reality* (London: Collins/Fontana Library,
1968), p. 88.

2. *Mahabharata* XII.318.7.

3. See the in-depth study by C. Pensa, "On the purification concept in Indian tradition, with special regard to Yoga," *East and West*, new series, XIX
(Rome, 1969).

4. *Yoga-Sutra* III.36–37.

CHAPTER 22

THE FINAL LEAP INTO TRANSCENDENCE

THE SUPRACONSCIOUS ECSTASY

The forms of ecstasy described in chapter 20 tax the intellect as well as the patience of anyone who has not personally experienced the paradoxical merging of subject and object, which is characteristic of these states. This is because the ecstatic consciousness occurs by definition only after the "brain" consciousness has been deactivated. That is to say, ecstasy ensues when the whirls of ordinary consciousness have been silenced through deep sensory inhibition, concentration, and meditation.

Nevertheless, as we have seen, it is wrong to assume that it is altogether impossible to make any reasonable assertions about these modalities of experience. The categoric statement that ecstasy, or mystical experience, is ineffable is only conditionally true. As R.M. Bucke, Alister Hardy, Marghanita Laski, and other researchers have demonstrated, it is quite possible to derive from descriptions of these experiences much valuable data.[1] The information they painstakingly gathered over many years has contributed greatly to our understanding of the evasive processes that take place in these states. In a way, the material presented on the previous pages corroborates the optimistic point of view that we can make sense of ecstasy.

The situation is somewhat different when we come to the type of ecstasy that lacks any form of object awareness. This is the condition known as "supraconscious ecstasy" (asamprajnata-samadhi) or "transconceptual ecstasy" (nirvikalpa-samadhi). Here it is no longer possible to draw information from any subjective experience, as this particular ecstatic state simply has no objective reference, or content.

The only concrete criterion at hand is the fact that the supra-

conscious ecstasy is devoid of any content. But what is consciousness without content? Stonelike unconsciousness?

This question already puzzled the ancient seers whose wisdom we encounter in the *Upanishads*. They correlated that rare
ecstatic state with the phenomenon of deep sleep, which is also
without object consciousness. In the *Brihad-Aranyaka-Upanishad*
(IV.3.19; 21), the nature of deep sleep is determined as follows:

> As a falcon or an eagle, having flown about there in space, be-
> comes fatigued, folds its wings, and repairs to its eyrie, just so
> the Spirit (purusha) hastens to that border[-state] where,
> asleep, it desires no desires and sees no dream [images].

> This is its essence in which, beyond [all] desires, it is free from
> sin and without fear. For, as one, when embraced by a beloved
> wife, is not conscious of what is within and without, so also
> this Spirit, embraced by awareness,[2] does not know what is
> within or without. This is its essence in which it is desire-ful-
> filled, desirous of the Self and [yet] without desire.

According to the explanation of the Vedanta teachers of antiquity, consciousness returns to the womb of transcendental Awareness in deep sleep. This return lacks an accompanying wakefulness, and the veil of spiritual blindness prevents the psyche from
coming to a genuine *unio mystica*.

In the *Vedanta-Paribhasha* (VII), the following definition is proffered for the altered state of consciousness called "deep sleep."

> [That which is] designated as "deep sleep" is a state [in which]
> a "whirl" of nescience is in the realm of nescience.

This definition is admittedly somewhat obscure. What it tries
to say is that deep sleep is a function of the fundamental spiritual
ignorance from which the unenlightened individual suffers. There
is no deep sleep for the enlightened being. He or she is always fully
awake, a *buddha*. Spiritual ignorance is operative also in the waking state, but in the case of deep sleep, consciousness returns to the
very matrix of spiritual nescience. Deep sleep is thus the state of
consciousness that is both nescient and latent.

In the *Mandala-Brahmana-Upanishad* (II.3.3–4) we read:

Even though there is similarity between sleep and ecstasy [in regard to] the dissolution of the mind [in both states], there is nonetheless a great difference between these two inasmuch as [sleep] is the absorption into *tamas* and is ineffective as a means for emancipation.

Upon the elimination of *tamas* in ecstasy . . . the dissolution of the phenomenal reality is achieved in the [supreme] Witness-Consciousness.

The phenomenal reality is said to be dissolved, because its representation in the empirical consciousness is eliminated in the ecstatic state. Thus the spiritual practitioner is effectively cut off from the external world. He or she has become the Witness-Consciousness (*sakshi-caitanya*), the transcendental Subject that apperceives all contents of consciousness, or their absence.

That the extinction of consciousness does not imply the loss of transcendental Awareness is argued in Vedanta from the fact that one "remembers" the absence of any contents of consciousness in deep sleep. Without the witnessing Awareness, the Self, this would be impossible. The continuous Self is the percipient of all modalities of consciousness.

As opposed to deep sleep, the translucent consciousness involution pursued in Yoga leads to a state that can be described as an awakening to Self-Awareness or, paradoxically, as waking sleep. The Indian nondualist schools speak of this state as the "Fourth" (*turiya* or *caturtha*). Strictly speaking, it is not a state of consciousness at all, but pure Being, or the transcendental substratum of the three empirical states of consciousness—namely, waking, dreaming, and sleeping. In his *Mandukya-Karika* (I.7), the adept Gaudapada refers to it as the "cessation of phenomenal existence," and "mere Self."

This Fourth is disclosed in supraconscious or transconceptual ecstasy. Here existence itself is transcended. To the ordinary consciousness, this frontier-crossing experience appears as a leap into a perfect void: a void that is not sheer nothingness but the nonexistence of the conditioned reality of space-time.

How do the Sanskrit texts see this ultimate stage of ecstatic realization? In Shankara's *Viveka-Cudamani* (362), we find this verse:

When the mind, "cooked" [i.e., purified and matured] through incessant practice, enters the Absolute, then ecstasy becomes devoid of [all] objectification (*vikalpa*) and brings about the realization of the essence of the innate nondual bliss [of the Self].

In his *Yoga-Sutra* (I.18), Patanjali puts it pithily thus:

The other [ecstasy, i.e., the supraconscious state] follows upon the practice of the cessation of awarenesses (*pratyaya*) [and consists only of] a residuum of activators.[3]

The *Yoga-Bhashya* (I.18) furnishes the following explanation of this obscure aphorism:

The higher [type] of dispassion is the means to the [supreme supraconscious ecstasy]. Since the practice with a "prop" [i.e., the various forms of conscious ecstasy] is unsuited as an instrument [of liberation], the nonobjective cessation of the [ecstatic] awareness is taken as a prop. And this [ecstasy] is devoid of objects. The unsupported consciousness accompanying this practice becomes as it were nonexistent.

We find that this explanation by Vyasa is still rather technical. What he appears to be saying is this: In supraconscious ecstasy, there is no regular object or idea to prop up the intensely focused consciousness. Rather, this ecstatic condition unfolds against the backdrop of the cessation of all conscious functions. The nonexercise of conscious activity coincides with the apparent evaporation of consciousness itself.

In the above-quoted passage, Vyasa makes another important point, namely that access to the supraconscious ecstasy cannot be gained through any yogic operations but only by means of inner surrender. He calls it "higher dispassion" (*para-vairagya*). Ordinary dispassion is directed at specific things, whereas higher dispassion is a resolute No to the cosmos at large. This is equivalent to the Christian *via negativa*.

ECSTATIC SUPRACONSCIOUSNESS AND THE UNCONSCIOUS

The ecstasy without object consciousness cannot be equated with a mere regression into the unconscious. This is evident from the fact that it is said to delete the activators, or subliminal tendencies, in the depth-consciousness. In other words, supraconscious ecstasy is responsible for a profound restructuring and transformation of the unconscious.

Of course, having been written many centuries before Freud, the scriptures of Hinduism, Buddhism, or Jainism do not employ the term "unconscious." Instead, they speak of several stages or degrees of consciousness. Hence it is far more correct to employ the term "depth-consciousness," which functions as a storehouse of the subliminal activators (samskara). More appropriately, the depth-consciousness *is* the totality of the subliminal traces of world experience.[4] Patanjali used the term "memory" to express the same idea.[5]

By the power of these hidden activators, the unenlightened individual is continually thrown out of the inner continuum, the Self, into external experiences. This congenital propensity for externalizing consciousness is most forcefully experienced during practices for concentration and meditative absorption, which are sustained efforts to render the mind blank. Of course, meditative blankness is not merely stupefaction. As Paul Brunton pointed out:

A mere emptiness of mind is not enough, is not the objective of these practices. Some idiots possess this naturally but they do not possess the wisdom of the Overself, the understanding of Who and What they are.[6]

If meditation is so difficult it is because it goes against the grain of our inner psychogenetic programming. For, by ingrained tendency, we are always casting our lot with the senses, and we are habitually uncentered. Meditation seeks to reveal to us our true identity. The mind must be made like a highly polished mirror so that the light of the Self can be reflected in it.

Only continued practice, which produces counteractive subliminal activators, can effectively block the tenacious program that inhibits our awareness of the Self. Persistence in meditation establishes the "consciousness of inversion" (*pratyak-cetana*).[7] The systematic involution of consciousness reaches its climax in the supraconscious ecstasy. Here the subliminal activators created by, and conducive to, the process of inversion gradually swallow up the entire stock of subliminal activators created by, and responsible for, the externalization of consciousness. These counteractive forces in the depth-consciousness become themselves used up during this process. When all latent deposits or "seeds" are thus consumed, liberation results. As the supraconscious ecstasy unfolds out of the ecstasy with objective prop, so liberation is the fruit of the ecstasy devoid of object consciousness and ideation. Liberation is the Self's appropriation of itself, or the person's awakening to his or her eternal freedom—a quite paradoxical event. At any rate, this step into the void of Being is thought to be final and irrevocable. It is the transcendence of all Becoming, or mystical death.

NOTES

1. See R.M. Bucke, *Cosmic Consciousness: A Study of the Evolution of the Human Mind* (Hyde Park, NY: University Books, 1961); A. Hardy, *The Spiritual Nature of Man: A Study of Contemporary Religious Experience* (Oxford: Clarendon Press, 1979); M. Laski, *Ecstasy: A Study of Some Secular and Religious Experiences* (Los Angeles: J.P. Tarcher, 1990).

2. The Sanskrit text has *prajna-atman*, which literally means "conscious Self," here rendered as "awareness." According to all spiritual traditions of Hinduism, awareness is the very essence of the transcendental Reality.

3. Previous translators have understood this aphorism differently.

4. The Yoga texts distinguish between *samskaras* and *vasanas*. The latter are the "trails" or patterns left behind in the depth-consciousness by our volitional activities, of which the samskaras can be said to be the individual constituents. As Vyasa puts it in his *Yoga-Bhashya* (IV.9): "The vasanas are the deposits of the activators."

5. See *Yoga-Sutra* IV.9.

6. P. Brunton, *Meditation* (Burdett, NY: Larson Publications, 1986), p. 134. This is volume 4 of *The Notebooks of Paul Brunton*.

7. See *Yoga-Sutra* I.29.

CHAPTER 23

THE GOAL: PERFECT ISOLATION

THE PATH OF REDUCTION TO THE SINGLE SELF

Orthodox Hindu ethics postulates four broad goals of human existence: material welfare (*artha*), cultural interests (*kama*), moral behavior (*dharma*), and liberation (*moksha*). Of these, the extrication from conditioned existence and the awakening to the ever-present reality of the Self is deemed the *summum bonum* of human life.

Liberation, or Self-realization, is the quintessence of all branches of Indian spirituality. Each tradition tries to realize this goal in its own distinct way.

The ascetics and sages realized early on that the intellect permeated by feelings, desires, and biases is ill-suited for lifting the veil that conceals the Reality behind phenomenal existence. In this respect they anticipated Immanuel Kant's critical speculations about the limits of the human mind in understanding reality. As Kant argued:

> It is true we cannot have a concept of what things may be in themselves beyond all possible experience.[1]

Kant, whose ideas brought about a Copernican revolution in Western philosophy, denied human beings the ability to see things as they are. He made metaphysical knowledge a matter of pure reason. By contrast, the great spiritual teachers of India without exception insisted that it is possible, through systematic discipline, to transcend the subject-object division peculiar to the intellect. For them, the human mind was indeed incapable of apprehending Reality. Yet, they also declared that the intellect was not the highest faculty of the psyche. They spoke of a transcendental mode of knowing, which they often called the "eye of gnosis" or "divine eye."[2]

Strictly speaking, however, this special form of wisdom can

not be labelled "knowledge" or "experience." Gnosis (*vidya*) is not just an act of knowledge. No subject or object is involved. It is a state of being. Hence the term "realization," in place of "cognition" or "knowledge," seems more appropriate to characterize this essentially transcognitive event.

Gnosis, in this context, is the apprehension of Reality as it is in itself, not as the human mind perceives it in the state of multiplicity. To "understand" what things are in themselves, one must assume their very nature by actually becoming them. This is achieved in the ontic identification of ecstasy (samadhi). In the ecstatic condition, as we have seen, consciousness coincides with the structure of the contemplated object. Thus the *Varaha-Upanishad* (II.18–23) states:

> The eye of gnosis beholds the all-pervasive Being-Awareness-Bliss. The eye of nescience does not see the Resplendent, just as a blind person [does not see] the sun. That Absolute, characterized by truth and awareness (*prajnana*), is awareness alone. It is only by thus fully knowing the Absolute that a mortal becomes immortal. Upon knowing for oneself that Bliss of the Absolute, which is nondual, devoid of opposites, filled with truth and awareness, one does not fear any form wherever. The position of the knowers of the Absolute is that clearly nothing exists but the Absolute alone, which is pure Awareness (*cit*), all-pervading, eternal, full, blissful, and imperishable. For the ignorant person the world is inundated with misery, whereas for the sage it is full of Bliss. To a blind person the world is dark, whereas for the clear-sighted it is bright.

Gnosis expresses a shift in consciousness and being. This chameleon process, difficult to understand intellectually, is founded on the fundamental axiom of spirituality that being and consciousness are not diametrically opposed entities, but complementary aspects or symbols of the one Reality. Wisdom is the immediate realization of the truth of this axiom.

While the lower forms of ecstasy, which are connected with an object, yield a special kind of knowing called *prajna*, the ultimate ecstatic state consists in the realization of the transintelligible Self.

The permanent actualization of Selfhood is known as liberation. All forms of samadhi disclose Reality, but only the ultimate, supraconscious type of ecstasy reveals the ultimate dimension of Reality, which is the Self. On the lower ecstatic levels, ontic identification with various layers of Nature occurs.

Since Reality comprises many levels, there is more than one "thing in itself," to borrow Kant's phrase. Most traditions recognize the Self, or Spirit, as the ultimate Thing. However, some theistic schools, such as Ramanuja's, regard the Self as an infinite, eternal "fragment" of the Divine. At any rate, India's spiritual traditions are all in agreement that the human being, though unable to intellectually know Reality in its nakedness, can *become* it in its different dimensions of totality.

While ecstatic identification with a given object of attention— be it coarse or subtle—is considered superior to mere intellectual knowledge, the most prized spiritual attainment of all is Self-realization itself.

LIBERATION AS ISOLATION

How does the goal of mythic spirituality present itself? All processes of spiritual unification, carried out on the physical and the mental level, are geared toward liberation. This is always conceived of as the antithesis of mundane or conditioned existence (*samsara*). For Patanjali and also for the followers of the Vaisheshika system, liberation means total isolation from the world: the discarding of all transient phenomena and the disentanglement even from the primary constituents of the created universe.

In other words, the fulfillment of mythic spirituality lies in the practitioner's absolute withdrawal from the phenomenal reality, in its visible and its invisible dimensions.

For this reason, King Bhoja was quite justified in defining the central activity of Yoga as one of "separation" (*viyoga*). Significantly, Patanjali chose the word *kaivalya* or "aloneness" to label the ultimate goal of his eightfold path. As the *Yoga-Sutra* (IV.34) states:

The resorption of the primary constituents [of Nature, which have become] devoid of purpose for the Self is [what is designated as] "aloneness," or the Power of Awareness abiding in [its] essence.

The "Power of Awareness" (*citi-shakti*) is, of course, the transcendental Self, the Witness of all consciousness processes or, as Kant would put it, the "transintelligible subject." Liberation is everything that conditioned existence is not: It is acausal, atemporal, aspatial, and unconditioned. An oft-cited passage in one of the Buddha's sermons has this:

> [Liberation is] the realm where there is neither earth nor water, neither fire nor air; not the realm of space-infinity, nor the realm of consciousness-infinity, nor the realm of no-thingness, nor the realm of neither-perception-nor-non-perception; neither this world nor a world yonder nor both, neither the sun nor the moon. Here, monks, I declare that there is no coming or going, no duration or destruction or origination. This is without support, without continuance, without condition. This is the end of suffering.[3]

This description of the state of "extinction" (nirvana) is admittedly atypical of the Pali canon. The Buddha was usually more reticent about metaphysical matters. Nonetheless, these presumably authentic words of the founder of Buddhism indicate that he did not conceive of extinction as mere nothingness.

The *Laghu-Yoga-Vasishtha* (VI.13.93a), which promulgates an idealistic metaphysics, also reminds us to be careful not to endow this uncreated state with anthropomorphous features:

> [That which] is called liberation is without location and without time. [Thus it is] not an ordinary state.

If liberation is not a state in the conventional sense of the term, it is also is not the creation of a new mode of existence. Rather, it is the recovery of the original wholeness, that is, the uncovering of the eternal purity of Reality. The Self is the same before and after the attainment of liberation. Human beings merely believe themselves to be fettered or freed. "Liberation," in other words, is as much a convention of speech as "bondage." The *Shvetashvatara-Upanishad* (II.14) puts it this way:

Even as a disc stained by dust shines brilliantly when cleansed, so the embodied [being], on seeing the reality of the Self, becomes unitary, fulfilled and free from sorrow.

Liberation is a simple switch of identity. Prior to liberation—from the unenlightened perspective—there is the thought of being a human being. Upon liberation, or enlightenment, this thought ceases. The Self knows itself to be the eternal Self, not a specific individual inhabiting a particular point in space and time.

Most schools teach that the act of liberation is final and irreversible. It follows upon the obliteration of all conditioned adjuncts. That is to say, liberation coincides with the complete decomposition of the body-mind on all levels of existence at the moment of death. All "bodies," or layers of apparent finite existence, are peeled away. Only the radiant nucleus, the Self, remains. At least this is the basic conviction of mythic spirituality.

Thus, in some schools of Vedanta, the abolition of the phenomenal entity is described as the transcendence of the five "sheaths" (*kosha*). These are conceived as veils around the eternal luminosity of the Self. In order of their density they are:

1. *anna-maya-kosha* — the physical body sustained by "food" (*anna*)

2. *prana-maya-kosha* — the body composed of vital force (*prana*), in Western occultism also known as the "etheric double"

3. *mano-maya-kosha* — the mental sheath, also referred to as the "astral body"

4. *vijnana-maya-kosha* — the sheath composed of knowledge

5. *ananda-maya-kosha* — the sheath consisting of pure bliss

These five sheaths, or fields, obscure the Self and hence are also called "superimpositions" (*upadhi*). They constitute the illusory reality experienced by unenlightened beings. In the *Panca-Dashi* (III.22), a Vedanta work of the fourteenth century, we read:

Upon the relinquishment of the five sheaths, [only] the Witness-Awareness [of the Self] remains.

This notion of "disembodied liberation" or *videha-mukti* is favored by, among others, the Vedanta teachers Ramanuja, Bhaskara, Yadava, Nimbarka, Sarvajnatma Muni, Prakashananda, Shri Kantha and Baladeva. It is also the viewpoint of the Nyaya and Vaisheshika schools of thought, as well as of Patanjali and Ishvara Krishna, the principal spokesman of Classical Samkhya.

This ideal contrasts with the alternative notion of "liberation in life" or *jivan-mukti*, which is based on the assumption that liberation is not a post-mortal affair but is realizable in this very life. This second view is put forward in the *Bhagavad-Gita*, the *Yoga-Vasishtha*, Shaiva Siddhanta, Mahayana Buddhism, and Vajrayana Buddhism, as well as by Shankara, Vidyaranya, and, in the twentieth century, by Sri Aurobindo.

LIBERATION: ONE OR MANY?

An important question arises here, namely whether liberation is the same in every case or whether the Buddhist nirvana, the Vedantic moksha, Patanjali's kaivalya and the brahma-nirvana of the *Bhagavad-Gita* denote different realizations. There is sufficient evidence to show that these designations are not merely linguistic variations. Each seems to have its own distinct meaning. This fact becomes strikingly obvious when one compares the concept of liberation in theistic schools with that of atheistic systems, such as Classical Samkhya. These differences were understood by the Indians themselves. For example, Srinivasadasa, in the seventeenth century, made the following highly relevant remark:

> Seekers of liberation are of two kinds: those who strive for *kaivalya* and those who strive for *moksha*. What is called *kaivalya* [is attained] through the Yoga of wisdom and consists in the realization of one's innate Self as distinct from Nature. This realization . . . is without the realization of the Lord.[4]

As opposed to this, moksha is said to be realized through loving attachment (bhakti) to God or through unconditional self- offering (*prapatti*). A careful analysis of the scriptures of other systems shows up further differentiations in the concepts of emancipation. Thus, it appears that the transcendental unity of all religions postulated by some historians of religion is a theological oversimplication.

At the same time, it is also true that these various concepts have a common denominator, namely the realization of a level of being that transcends the ordinary space-time continuum. But this must not blind us to the equally significant distinctions. The evidence suggests that there are actual nuances in the state of liberation, as realized by the adherents of diverse schools. Moreover, it would seem plausible that these nuances are in fact degrees of completeness of realization.

LIBERATION THROUGH GRACE

All the spiritual traditions of India emphasize that liberation cannot be "achieved" or "procured," but it buds as its own cause. This notion has led the theistic thinkers of Yoga to formulate the doctrine of grace (prasada). Possibly the earliest mention of this theological teaching is in the *Katha-Upanishad* (II.20):

He who is devoid of [selfish] will and free from sorrow, beholds through the grace of the Creator the magnanimity of the Self.

Three stanzas later, the same scripture states:

This Self cannot be attained by instruction, nor by the intellect, nor by much listening [to the Vedic lore]. This [Self] is attained by him whom it chooses. To him this Self reveals its form (*tanu*).[5]

The concept of grace is in a certain sense a personification of the wholly transcendental act of recovering the autonomy of Selfhood. To the finite mind the event of liberation presents itself as having been initiated by the Divine Being. The *Vishnu-Purana* (VI.7.30) has this pertinent verse:

That Absolute, O sage, verily attracts the contemplator [who has reached] the state of the Self, as a magnet attracts [metal] by its own power and [that of its magnetized] products.

Even such a staunch nondualist as Shankara, who reinterpreted

Upanishadic passages to avoid speaking of grace, admitted:

> . . . the apprehension of the Absolute is not dependent on human activity. What then? [It is] dependent on the Thing itself [i.e., the Absolute].[6]

Reason fails to comprehend this ultimate mystery. Liberation, however it may be conceived, is paradoxical. The schools most expressive of the mythic consciousness indirectly seek to reduce this paradox by making liberation a state to be realized apart from the world and the body-mind. It is truly a condition of isolation, but an isolation that consists in infinite Awareness and Bliss at the level of the most generic existence, which is that of the transcendental Reality.

The ideal of liberation in life represents a more integral point of view, which combines Self-realization with conditioned existence. One eye is firmly fixed on the Infinite, the other gazes at the world of change. There is not merely ascent to the spiritual dimension but also the descent of the Spirit into matter, or conscious participation by the Spirit in the evolution of individuated life. We will encounter this great realization of wholeness in Part Two of this book.

NOTES

1. R. Schmidt, ed., *Immanuel Kant—Die drei Kritiken* (Stuttgart: Kroner Taschenbuch, 1960), pp. 150–151.

2. The respective Sanskrit terms are *jnana-cakshus* and *divya-cakshus*. See, for instance, the *Bhagavad-Gita* (XI.8), the *Atma-Bodha* (47), and the *Amrita-Bindu-Upanishad* (21).

3. *Udana* 80.

4. *Yatindra-Mata-Dipika* VIII.16.

5. See also *Mundaka-Upanishad* III.2.3.

6. *Brahma-Sutra-Bhashya* I.1.4.

CHAPTER 24

IN RETROSPECT: THE SPIRITUALITY OF SHIVA

THE WORLD-RENOUNCING MYSTICS AND SAGES

In the chapters so far, we have examined in some depth the basic features of the mythic strand of spirituality in India. It seems appropriate now to review some of the focal points that have been identified.

First of all, mythic spirituality is exclusively oriented toward transcendence. This propensity to otherworldliness manifests itself in the consistent attempt to exit from our space-time universe. Psychologically, this finds expression in a prominent striving for unification and simplification, until the One, the Simplex, beyond all plurality and complexity is reached.

Sociologically, the mythic vector toward transcendence shows itself in the strong trend to opt out of social life, which involves the abandoning of family, work, and communal responsibilities.

A collateral expression of this extreme individualistic attitude is a general devaluation of the body, which is considered as the seat of all evil and at best as an "open sore" or "monstrous wound" needing attention.[1] This is tied in with a marked denigration of the female gender, which is regarded as a capital source of temptation and spiritual degradation.

The aspirants of mythic spirituality seek hermetic insulation from the external environment in order to be able to empty their inner world completely and create in themselves a vacuum that will allow them to cross the threshold into the dimension of pure Being. Everything that removes attention from this central task is seen as a temptation and obstruction.

The meditative path of mythic spirituality can be regarded as a technique for achieving voluntary death. According to the *Chandogya-Upanishad* (VI.8.6), at the moment of death the senses enter the mind, which, in turn, merges into the life force. This, again, becomes radiant light and flows into the supreme Godhead, thus effecting a total disintegration of the empirical entity. In the view of the nondualist metaphysics of Vedanta, the individual *becomes* the Absolute.

However, in the case of an ordinary mortal this coincidence with the Absolute is not achieved consciously and hence has no salvific power. After a certain period, the individual's residual karma leads to incarnation in one of the levels of conditioned existence. Only duly prepared spiritual adepts enter, after the demise of the body, the Absolute with full awareness. This secures for them permanent liberation from the "wheel of becoming," the world of change, uncertainty, anxiety, and sorrow.

Mythic spirituality is the path of the renunciate (*samnyasin*) who has left everything behind; the ascetic (*tapasvin, yati*) who spares no pains to transcend the world of suffering; the *yogin* who strives to escape the state of "disunion" (*viyoga*); the Buddhist *arahant* who in his solitary sojourn through the world is compared to the single horn of a rhinoceros; and the Vedic *muni* who, in his ecstasy, beholds the world from on high.

The muni is of particular interest. The word itself means "he who practices silence" and was, significantly enough, also used as an honorific title for Gautama the Buddha. Just as vocal expression is the most outstanding characteristic of the mythic structure of consciousness (the Greek verb *mytheomai* means "to speak"), so silence or *mauna* is wholly magical. Silence is a sacred and sacralizing act. It is intimately connected with the concept of numinous power. Those who are silent conserve their life force and gain access to the sacred and its power.

Silence is possibly the oldest form of ascetic discipline. It was widely enjoyed by the early Vedic priests, for only silence could reveal the mysterious sound that permeates the universe—*om*. Even today the teachers of some yogic traditions express their consent to accept a pupil by silence.

SHIVA—SYMBOL OF NEGATION AND INTEGRATION

The temper of mythic spirituality is captured most impressively in the image of Shiva, the God *par excellence* of the yogins.

Shiva is a chthonic deity and as such is connected with death, ancestor worship, and rebirth. He wears a third eye in the middle of
his forehead, representing his tremendous spiritual power. With
this eye he sees into the hearts of all beings and also sends out his
death-bringing rays to punish the wicked.

Lord Shiva is commonly depicted with the few utensils of a
wandering ascetic with disheveled hair. He wanders about naked,
covering his body from toe to crown with ashes. His skin color is
blue, suggesting his dominion over the subtle dimensions of existence. His favorite dwelling place is the cemetery or cremation
ground, and he wears a necklace of skulls. His special emblem is
the serpent as the symbol of regeneration and rebirth, but also of
death and the venomousness of mundane existence.

In the Puranas, the orthodox priests are said to have hated
Shiva for his disregard of the established social order. They saw
him not as a benign (*shiva*) being but as an immodest and malevo-
lent divinity.

Yet, there is another side to Shiva, which brings home the fact
that he *is* divine and therefore utterly paradoxical. For, despite all
his terrifying asceticism, Shiva is no stranger to passion. He has a
genuine Dionysian aspect. Together with his divine spouse
Parvati, he is said to reside at the peak of Kailasa, the world mountain. There the couple enjoys continuous sexual union, which releases great Bliss. Thus Shiva is the arch-Tantric. His numerous
sexual exploits with demigods and humans are all part of his divine play. His intense eroticism suggests that ascetics are not feeble
eunuchs but beings endowed with great power. Shiva's seed is
said to destroy those who are not spiritually prepared to receive it.

Shiva's paradoxical character, which combines transcendence
and eroticism, points toward a more integral perspective. Thus,
theological imagination has accomplished what social practice
failed to achieve: the integration of opposites. Upon the figure of
Shiva we find projected all those aspects of existence that the traditions of mythic spirituality stringently exclude from their quest for
the One. Only the Lord can be both fierce ascetic and sinner. The
ordinary mortal aspiring to transcendence must shun all the out-
bursts of passion for which Shiva is notorious.

In the practice of mythic spirituality, no compromise with the world is possible. Male ascetics cannot also be seducers of women, and female aspirants cannot also enjoy marital bliss. The longed-for exodus from the universe is possible only through the radical renunciation of all typically human self-expressions. The mythic aspirants limit themselves to reach the Unlimited. The Divine alone transcends even this limitation.

As we will see, only in the more integral spiritual traditions, like certain schools of Tantrism, have spiritual practitioners dared to model their lives directly after the paradoxical Divine. They sought to integrate worldly existence with their spiritual aspirations.

NOTE

1. See V. Trenckner, *Milindapanha* (London: Royal Asiatic Society, 1928), p. 73.

PART TWO

INTEGRAL ASPECTS OF SPIRITUALITY

HE FROM WHOM THE WORLD DOES NOT RECOIL
AND WHO DOES NOT RECOIL FROM THE WORLD,
WHO IS RELEASED FROM THRILL-SEEKING,
IMPATIENCE, AND FEAR, IS SAID TO BE
LIBERATED IN LIFE.

VARAHA-UPANISHAD IV.3.26

CHAPTER 25

FROM TRANSCENDENCE TO WHOLENESS

MYTHIC INWARDNESS AND THE AESTHETIC PROCESS

Mythic spirituality, as we have seen, is the unreserved delving into the depths of the psyche, combined with a systematic withdrawal from the external world. It is the embodiment of the urge to transcend the immediately given, the tangible realm, in favor of the formless Infinite.

Paradoxically, this urge toward unity and transcendence finds its most tangible manifestation in the plastic art of India. The sculptures of the temples and other sacred places are the mythic unifying impulse made palpable. When we examine the great temple sculptures, we find that Gods and saints are characteristically depicted with full, round bodies. The images have an almost sensuous quality. In view of the prevalent ascetical orientation, we would expect to find portrayals of emaciated figures, but these are rare.

The reason for this is that the sculptures seldom represent the physical human body but generally mean to convey something of the rotundness of the subtle body, which mystics experience as a cloak of energy surrounding the material form. Depictions of male and female deities, with many arms and sometimes many heads, clearly do not belong to the material world. What some art historians have described as effeminate is in effect an effort to depict the androgynous nature of the Divine.

But even portrayals of ascetics and sages, seated cross-legged or standing upright, with hands carefully positioned in appropriate gestures (mudra) and eyes shut or wide open in ecstasy, are windows onto the hidden dimension. This is as true of Hindu art as it is of Jaina and Buddhist iconography. As A.L. Basham observed:

Asceticism and self-denial in various forms are praised in

much Indian religious literature, but the ascetics who appear in sculpture are usually well fed and cheerful. As an example we may cite the colossal rock-cut medieval image of the Jaina saint Gommatesvara at Sravana Belgola in Mysore. He stands bolt upright in the posture of meditation known as *kayotsarga*, with feet firm on the earth and arms held downwards but not touching the body, and he smiles faintly. The artist must have tried to express the soul almost set free from the trammels of matter, and about to leave for its final resting place of everlasting bliss at the top of the universe.[1]

The yogic origin of these artistic creations is undeniable. In India, the artist is in fact called *yogin* and *sadhaka* ("realizer"). It is by means of concentration, meditation, visualization, and other well-tried techniques of Yoga that he penetrates into the innermost essence of the idea he intends to depict. This applies to the sculptor as much as to the painter and poet. Sculpture, painting, and verse must first have matured to full reality in the mind of the artist before he can set out to express them concretely.

In other words, the external act of shaping the work of art is merely a reproduction of the finished artistic creation in the consciousness of the artist. A fitting example for this is Valmiki's *Ramayana* epic whose complex story is said to have first been experienced mentally and then transcribed into written language. Similarly, India's other great national epic, the *Mahabharata*, is celebrated as the work of the sage Vyasa. Tradition has it that he dictated the entire composition of more than 100,000 verses to the elephant-headed God Ganesha, who alone was fast enough to follow the dictation.

Unlike the artist, however, the aspirant of mythic spirituality is not concerned with projecting outward what he or she experiences within. On the contrary, these practitioners see no good in communication and therefore typically seal themselves off from society, setting their heart on reaching ever deeper levels of inwardness.

Besides, the internal creative activity of yogins cannot properly be equated with the aesthetic process. Artistic visualization is an entirely positive event resulting in a concrete work. By contrast, the spiritual practitioners aspire to the complete negation of all forms or concepts in nirvikalpa-samadhi, the transconceptual ecstasy. This strictly otherwordly orientation has its modern parallel in Theravada Buddhism, many of whose adherents go as far as to decry aesthetic experience as being antagonistic to the path of unification.

ASCETICAL AND HOLISTIC TRENDS IN INDIA

More often than not, the life-denying *via negativa* is held to be representative of the whole of Indian culture. This is decidedly not the case, however. When we look more closely at the cultural history of India, we notice a process of tension between two equally powerful trends: the one otherwordly or ascetic and the other syncretistic or holistic. Sometimes these cultural streams have been called "cathartic" and "hedonistic" respectively, but these terms are far too loaded to be useful. The concepts of transcendence and wholeness, proposed in this volume, do better justice to the complex evolutionary forces that have woven the rich tapestry of Indian civilization.

Both transcendence-oriented and integral teachings have coexisted from very early times and have mutually enriched, modified, and complemented each other. The purely ascetic or renunciatory (*shramana*) current, as it manifests itself with full vigor in older Buddhism, Jainism, Classical Yoga, and Advaita Vedanta, certainly belongs to the mythic structure of consciousness.[2] By contrast, the more syncretistic philosophies as expressed, for instance, in the *Bhagavad-Gita*, Mahayana Buddhism, and Tantrism, contain distinctly recognizable integral features.

The earliest *Upanishads*, which were composed in the eighth and ninth century B.C. or perhaps earlier still, offer us glimpses of the struggle between the ascetic and the more holistic orientations in India's complex civilization. The Upanishadic sages taught two great secret doctrines. The first is the occult teaching of karma and rebirth (punar-janman), and the second is the ideal of liberation (moksha). The latter endorsed the pursuit of asceticism not as an instrument of attaining worldly goods, such as health, wealth, and happiness, but as a means of transcending mundane existence itself.

These innovative teachings were promptly institutionalized by the orthodox priests in the model of the four stages of life, called ashramas.[3] In turn, their two main contributions to the emerging Hindu society were the caste system on one hand and the Sanskrit language on the other.

The chief stimulators and bearers of this formidable synthesis were two religious communities at the fringe of the Vedic orthodoxy, namely the Vratya brotherhoods dedicated to the worship of the God Rudra-Shiva and the large circle of Vishnu devotees. In both religious camps, Yoga was an important practice. The striking difference between these two traditions is that the Vratyas espoused the ascetic approach, whereas the Vaishnava community combined a healthy interest in mundane life with the newly discovered ideal of liberation.

The remarkable Pancaratra tradition, an early form of Vaishnavism, bears eloquent witness to this integral orientation.[4] The grand sacred scripture of this important cultural current is the *Bhagavad-Gita* ("Song of the Lord"). Besides being a religious classic and possibly the only truly philosophical poem in the world, this text documents that early unparalleled effort to achieve a creative synthesis between renunciation and world-affirmation, leading to the formulation of the ideal of *loka-samgraha*, which is the spiritual transformation of the world.

The crucial existential problem taken up in the *Bhagavad-Gita* is the question of the relationship between individual religiosity and social obligations, or how to render unto God what is God's and unto Caesar what is Caesar's. Thus, we may regard this work as the first full-fledged holistic manifestation of the Indian mind.

A second unique integral breakthrough occurred almost a millennium later with the emergence of Tantrism in the first centuries A.D. The Tantric movement, which swept over the entire Indian subcontinent, was the culmination of the long osmosis between Vedic Brahmanism, the popular religious cults, and the native non-Sanskritic Indian traditions.

The distinction between the world-affirmative attitude of the ancient Vedic culture and the ascetic orientation, which flourished at its margins, can best be illustrated in their different interpretations of the well-known virtue of nonharming (ahimsa).

According to the *Rig-Veda* and the Mimamsa school, which is the most orthodox philosophical system of Brahmanism, the moral imperative of nonharming does not extend to the ritual slaughtering of animals. This view is diametrically opposed to the ideal of nonharming put forward by the strictly ascetic traditions, which demand that it be applied universally. From the ascetic perspective, the Vedic injunction to take the life of animals for sacrificial purposes is karmic and therefore detrimental to the attainment of true freedom.

The ascetic ideal of absolute nonharming was given its most radical expression in Jainism. Even Buddhism forbids the slaughter of creatures, and this ideal also was preserved in the Mahayana and Vajrayana Buddhist schools.

Because of the considerable control exercised by the Vedic orthodoxy, mainstream Hinduism always worked on compromise solutions to check the radical ascetic mode with its demand for unqualified nonviolence. This moderate attitude is characteristic of the *Mahabharata*, the Puranas, and the juridical literature, as well as the *Bhagavad-Gita*.

In fact, the philosophical discourse between the God-man Krishna and the hero Arjuna, which forms the dramatic framework of the "Lord's Song", concerns the lawfulness of some wars. After a long and twisted argument, Krishna finally convinces his princely disciple that it is perfectly justifiable, and even necessary, to wage war against those who seek to uproot the spiritual principles of existence.

Vyasa, the main commentator of the *Yoga-Sutra*, proposed a similar ethics of compromise. He distinguished between the "great vow" (*maha-vrata*) of the ascetics for whom nonharming is unconditional and the "minor vow" (*anu-vrata*) of lay persons who may commit harm (*himsa*) within the scope of their profession, as sanctioned by their particular tradition.[5] Thus, it is incumbent on a soldier to protect his country, if necessary, by violent means.

For we who have witnessed the devastation of two world wars and live under the threat of a possible nuclear holocaust, the pacifist philosophies of Mahatma Gandhi, Martin Luther King, and the present Dalai Lama are likely to hold greater appeal than the caste-bound moral teachings of the *Bhagavad-Gita* or the *Maha-*

bharata. Nevertheless, within the context of Indian civilization, we must acknowledge that they are in fact gesturing toward a more integral view of life.

The millennia-long struggle that has taken place between the world-affirmative and the world-denying attitudes in India is strikingly portrayed in the following episode in the *Mahabharata* (IX.50) epic.

Asita Devala was a faithful follower of the Vedic moral code. He was entirely devoted to virtue, chastity, and ascetic discipline. One day the yogin Jaigishavya arrived at Asita's hermitage and there settled down to continue with his advanced practices. Asita watched that great ascetic with keen interest, never leaving him out of sight for long and serving him unflaggingly. Yet for many years Jaigishavya did not utter a single sound of approval or disapproval.

Asita Devala grew increasingly perturbed and anxious. One day, while in meditation, he saw his illustrious and mysterious guest ascend to the celestial regions. Endowed with some spiritual gifts of his own, Asita pursued the yogin in his inner vision but, after having traversed many different realms, suddenly lost track of Jaigishavya. He had soared to ever higher spheres of existence, until he reached the supreme state of the Absolute itself.

Unable to follow, Asita brought his consciousness back to Earth, and on regaining his ordinary awareness he discovered to his great astonishment that Jaigishavya was sitting happily in his hermitage. Asita fell at the adept's feet. He begged him for instruction in the doctrine of liberation, solemnly affirming his readiness to renounce the world. Jaigishavya consented.

However, on hearing Asita Devala's firm resolve, the forefathers in the "realm of the ancestors" (*pitri-loka*), who had been sustained by his conscientious daily sacrifices, began to lament. They appeared before him, begging him to desist from this undertaking lest they should experience hunger and wither away without their daily sacrificial offerings.

Overwhelmed by pity for his ancestors, Asita Devala decided to abandon his resolution to dedicate himself entirely to the goal of liberation and instead to continue his way of life as an ordinary householder. Alas, he could not help wondering whether he had made the right choice. Then, on second thought, he turned back to his previous resolve, devoted himself to the ideal of renunciation, and in due course obtained the eternal freedom of the Self.

NOTES

1. A.L. Basham, *The Wonder that was India: A Survey of the History and Culture of the Indian Sub-Continent before the Coming of the Muslims* (London: Fontana/Collins, 1971), p. 349.

2. The Indian scholar M. Sahay put forward the view that the Yoga of Patanjali has a world-oriented emphasis. He suggested that Patanjali valued the conscious ecstasy more than the supraconscious ecstasy (asamprajnata-samadhi). This is quite unfounded. There can be little question that Classical Yoga belongs to the mythic orientation. See M. Sahay, "Patanjala-Yogasutras and the Vyasa-Bhasya: An Examination," *Vishveshvaranand Indological Journal*, vol. 2 (1964), pp. 254–260.

3. The four stages of life are: pupilage, householder life, forest life, and final renunciation or total dedication to the ideal of spiritual liberation.

4. See O. Schrader, *Introduction to the Pancharatra and the Ahirbudhnya-Samhita* (Adyar, India: Theosophical Publishing House, 1916), 2 vols.

5. See *Yoga-Bhashya* II.31.

CHAPTER 26

THE YOGIN ON THE BATTLEFIELD

THE GRAND SYNTHESIS OF THE BHAGAVATA RELIGION

One of the most auspicious and far-reaching events in the cultural history of India was the emergence of the Pancaratra or Bhagavata religion. It was a major factor in the process of amalgamation leading to what is known today as Hinduism. The most incisive contributions of the Bhagavata religion were the introduction of pictorial worship, the erection of temples, the abstention from animal sacrifices, and the doctrine of multiple "incarnations" (*avatara*) of the Divine.

At the heart of this imposing syncretistic movement is the *Bhagavad-Gita*, which is celebrated as the sacred revelation of the Lord (*bhagavan*). Probably composed in the fourth or fifth century B.C., this scripture gives voice to still more ancient traditions. Yet it is a first unique effort to formulate a more integral view of life. Not surprisingly, the *Gita* ("Song"), as this Sanskrit work is widely called, has for generation after generation enjoyed immense popularity. It has even inspired many seer-bards to compose similar metaphysical songs, bearing the name *Gita*.[1]

The profound significance of the *Bhagavad-Gita* lies in the fact that it mediates between the this-worldly orientation and the ascetic transcendentalist trend. The shortcoming of the former attitude is its overemphasis of the exigencies of the visible universe, whereas the imperfection of the latter is its belittlement of mundane existence. In the *Gita* both orientations are brought together and integrated. Thus it avoids both the extreme of worldly magism and the extreme of otherworldly mysticism.

Even though the *Bhagavad-Gita* purports to represent a path of liberation, it eschews any form of escapism by insisting that the great goal can be realized amidst the manifold concerns of daily life. We need not forsake the world to find peace and enlightenment. On the contrary, we must find the Divine in the turmoil of life, in our every action.

THE DIVINE FULLNESS AND ETHICAL ACTIVISM

The ethical activism of the *Bhagavad-Gita* can be explained by reference to its theology. God Vishnu is conceived and worshipped as the ultimate, all-embracing Whole. He is both the "highest being" (*purusha-uttama*), the source of all creation, and the pulse of life beating in all things. He is neither, as in Judaism and Christianity, towering above his creatures in splendid isolation, nor is he merely identical with Nature, which is the contention of pantheist philosophers like Spinoza.

The position of the *Bhagavad-Gita* and of the Bhagavata religion in general is as follows: The created universe in its incomprehensible vastness rests in the Divine and in essence is of one nature with it, but the world does not limit or exhaust the Divine in the least. God is not purely transcendental Being, but is transcendental as well as immanent. He encompasses both Being and Becoming. Though reaching infinitely beyond the manifest reality, he is nonetheless innate in it and sustaining it. As Lord Krishna, the incarnate Divine, declares in the *Bhagavad-Gita* (IX.4–5):

> By Me, unmanifest in form, this entire [world] was spread out. All beings abide in Me, but I do not subsist in them.

> Nevertheless, beings do *not* abide in Me. Behold My lordly Yoga: My Self sustains [all] beings, yet not abiding in beings, causes beings to be.

Elsewhere (IX.16–18) Krishna states:

> I am the rite. I am the sacrifice. I am the oblation. I am the herb. I am the mantra. I am the ghee. I am the fire. I am the offering.

> I am the father of this world, the mother, the supporter, the grandsire, [everything that is] to be known, the purifier, the syllable *om*, and the *Rig-*, *Sama-*, and *Yajur-*[*Veda*].

> I am the course, the sustainer, the lord, witness, home and refuge, friend, origin, dissolution and the middle-state [of the

world], the treasure-house, the imperishable seed [in all beings].

The Divine is the perfect plenum (*purna*), of which a well-known Sanskrit verse says:

The Whole is that. The Whole is this. From the Whole the Whole is derived. The Whole taken from the Whole, the Whole [still] remains.

This metaphysical view cannot be subsumed under the headings of either deism or pantheism. If a label is required at all, it would have to be pan-en-theism. This Greek-derived term means "all-in-God-ism." It is perhaps the most congenial transcription of the Sanskrit compound *sharira-sharira-bhava*, which is the name of the theological doctrine that God's relationship to the finite world is analogous to the connection between mind and body.[2]

ACTION AND THE TRANSCENDENCE OF KARMA

The activistic tenor of the *Gita*'s teaching finds its symbolic expression in the fact that traditionally this didactic dialogue was delivered on the morning of one of the fiercest battles fought on Indian soil: the war between the Kauravas and the Pandavas. The former had usurped the latter's kingdom by trickery, and, having failed to regain the throne by peaceful means, the five sons of Pandu were now ready to fight for their inheritance and to restore order to the country.

Arjuna, one of the Pandava princes, had chosen the God-man Krishna for his charioteer. His enemies had slighted the wise Krishna and chosen instead a huge army armed to the teeth. Yet, the outcome of the war was predestined. Krishna, playing the role of divine trickster, proved a being not only of great wisdom but also cunning. Once he had convinced Arjuna of the necessity of a just war, the battle unfolded according to a divine plan. The Pandavas won back their kingdom, and the country flourished again under their benign rulership.

The battlefield, known as the *kuru-kshetra* ("field of the Kurus"), is thought to be located in the region of modern Delhi. However, it is clear from the *Gita* itself that this arena of bloodshed early on came to symbolize the battleground of life. It stands especially for the strife between good and evil, right and wrong.

The dialogue between Krishna and his disciple Arjuna in the *Gita* revolves around a very concrete problem: Is war always sinful? Or are there situations that demand and justify aggression? This question harbors a much more comprehensive philosophical issue: Does action redound to liberation?

According to the mythic tradition of asceticism, any action sullies human beings and necessarily leads to ever new sorrow and increased entanglement in the world. Action can never extricate them from the wheel of finite existence. The *Bhagavad-Gita* goes a completely new way in interpreting the metaphysical consequences of human activity. Krishna, the divine teacher, points out one irrefutable fact: To be alive means to act. Existence is incessant and interminable activity. Even the Divine itself is constantly dynamic, yet without forfeiting its simultaneous status as the imperturbable Witness of events:

> Not even for a moment can anyone ever remain without performing action. Everyone is unwittingly made to act by the constituents (guna) born of Nature (prakriti). (III.5)

> For Me, O son of Pritha [i.e., Arjuna], there is nothing to be done in the three worlds, nothing ungained to be gained—and yet I engage in action.

> For, if I were not untiringly ever to abide in action, people would, O son of Pritha, follow everywhere My "track" [i.e., My example].

> If I were not to perform actions, these worlds would perish, and I would be the author of chaos, destroying all these creatures. (III.22–24)

If even the Divine is constrained to act, how can we as human beings ever hope to attain to that sublime enlightenment that is the ultimate meaning and fulfillment of life? How can we escape from sorrowful existence? Krishna instructs Prince Arjuna in the two paths to liberation:

> Of yore I proclaimed a twofold way in this world, O guileless one: the Yoga of gnosis (*jnana-yoga*) for followers-of-Samkhya

and the Yoga of action (*karma-yoga*) for yogins. (III.3)

The Yoga of gnosis is the path of contemplative ascetics who seek enlightenment by withdrawing from mundane life and by cultivating higher knowledge in the solitude of the forest or mountain cave. The Yoga of action, in contrast, is suited for the active person, who chooses to live in the world. Both paths lead to the supreme goal, but the Yoga of action is said to be more excellent and complete.[3]

Even though external renunciation is not wrong in itself, it nevertheless negates one aspect of the Whole, namely the dynamism of life. Yet, our individual life must be understood as an aspect of the universal Life. Krishna emphatically declares the profound meaningfulness and intrinsic value of life. In doing so he overcomes the mythic conception of existence, which devalues individuated existence.

The spiritual path advocated and extolled by Krishna is founded on the principle of *inner* renunciation. Action can defile a person only so long as he or she performs it out of selfish motives and clings anxiously to its fruit:

Not by abstention from actions does a man enjoy action-transcendence (*naishkarmya*), nor by renunciation alone does he approach perfection. (III.4)

Therefore always perform unattached the right deed, for the man who performs action without attachment attains to the Supreme. (III.19)

Krishna continues:

What is action? What is inaction? About this even the sages are bewildered. I shall tell you that action which, once understood, will set you free from ill.

Indeed, one ought to understand [the nature] of action and one ought to understand wrong action (*vikarman*), and one ought to understand inaction (*akarman*). Impenetrable is the way of action.

He who sees inaction in action and action in inaction, is wise among men, yoked and performing whole actions.

He whose every enterprise is free from desire and motive and whose action is burned in the fire of wisdom, the wise call "learned" (*pandita*).

Having cast off [all] attachment to the fruit of actions, ever content, independent, though engaged in [right] action, he does not act at all.

Hoping for nothing, self and thought restrained, abandoning all possessions, performing action only with the body, he does not accumulate guilt. (IV.16–21)

Our actions become pure when we renounce the self, or ego, which is the source of moral defilement. We must step behind our work and be concerned only with what appears necessary in a given situation. Thus we are able to perform all action as unselfish sacrifice. This is the ideal of *naishkarmya-karman* or "actionless action," which is perhaps better translated as "action transcendence." This virtue corresponds to the Taoist practice of *wu wei*, as expressed in Lao Tzu's *Tao Te King* (37.1a):

The everlasting Tao does not act (*wu wei*).
And yet: nothing remains undone.

The same idea is expressed in another verse (48.1):

By pursuing learning, one increases daily.
By pursuing the Tao, one decreases daily.
One decreases and continues to decrease
until one arrives at not doing (*wu wei*).
Not doing, and yet: nothing remains undone.

Krishna makes it clear that "not doing" is not merely inactivity. He says:

In action alone is your rightful interest (*adhikara*), never in its fruits. Let not your motive be the fruit of action, nor let your attachment be to inaction.

Steadfast in Yoga, perform actions abandoning attachment, O Dhanamjaya, remaining the same in success and failure. Yoga is called balance (*samatva*). (II.47–48)

In the Yoga of action, the practitioner tries to emulate the para-doxical condition of the Divine, which is the harmonious integra-tion of activity and inactivity: God as creator and as transcendental witness. Yet, it would be a mistake to assume that the attitude of inner distance in the performance of actions is the sole criterion. For this would ignore the moral character of an act and indirectly sanction sinful deeds detrimental to the attainment of liberation.

An act must not only be done in a spirit of unselfishness, it must also be admissible in its content. In this context, Krishna em-ploys the term *karya*, meaning "that which is to be done," express-ing the ethical "ought."

To be precise, action must reflect, preserve, and promote the great moral order (dharma) in the universe. The concept of dharma is central to all philosophical traditions of India. This San-skrit word is derived from the verbal root *dhri*, meaning "to hold." Thus, dharma signifies the universal harmony that safeguards and directs the smooth flow of cosmic activity, and that manifests in each being as innate law (*sva-dharma*). Then again, dharma stands for the objective ethical norms, the mores and laws of the land, which are supposed to mirror the universal order.

The fulfillment of the objective law coincides, in principle, with the fulfillment of the innate law as it manifests in individual beings. This implies that in the *Bhagavad-Gita*, dharma must not exclusively be identified with the "unalterable customary order of class-duties or caste-duties and the general approved course of conduct for the people," as one historian of religion has proposed.[4] For such a view pays no heed to the profound psychological and metaphysical implications of that polymorphous concept.

Sva-dharma, again, is the law of active self-determination, the "ought" presented to our mind from deep within, so that our in-most being (*sva-bhava*) can fulfill itself. Sva-dharma is cognate with Socrates' concept of the *daimonion*, the inner voice, rather than with moral obligations embodied in certain external rules.

The *Gita* does not, of course, dispense with all authority. It is evident that those who have not yet penetrated to the clarity of sva-dharma are in need of moral guidance, as provided by tradi-tional law and the exemplary conduct of enlightened sages. However, those men and women are at the same time encouraged to develop their own consciences. Mere reliance on external rules is not enough.

Although the Sanskrit language lacks a precise synonym for "conscience," we find that the concept is contained in the more comprehensive term of the "wisdom-faculty" (buddhi), or enlightened reason. Once this higher organ of judgement is operative, we see the grand universal order within the compass of our own being and then become independent of external injunctions. As Krishna states:

> The *buddhi*-yoked leaves behind here [in this world] both good and evil. (II.50)

Without the awakening of the wisdom-faculty, the Self cannot be realized. Understandably, the kindling of the wisdom-faculty is therefore praised as the most precious goal to which a person can dedicate himself or herself. In the words of the God-man Krishna:

> Abandoning in thought all actions to Me, intent on Me, resorting to *buddhi-yoga*, be constantly Me-minded.

> Me-minded, you will transcend all obstacles by My grace. But if out of ego-sense (*ahamkara*) you will not listen, [then] you will perish! (XVIII.57–58)

There are three types of wisdom-faculty, depending on the predominance of the one or the other of the three primary constituents of Nature:

> The wisdom-faculty that understands activity and cessation, right and wrong, fear and fearlessness, bondage and liberation—that, O son of Pritha, is *sattva*-natured.

> The wisdom-faculty by which one knows norm and normlessness, right and wrong, not as [they really are]—that, O son of Pritha, is *rajas*-natured.

> The wisdom-faculty that, enveloped in darkness, thinks that normlessness is the norm and [that sees] all things [thus] reversed—that, O son of Pritha, is *tamas*-natured. (XVIII.30–32)

Krishna distinguishes between two grades of attainment in Yoga: the aspirant who is on the way to freedom and the adept who has reached the apex. They each follow their own particular mode of conduct:

> For the sage desiring to ascend [to the heights of] Yoga, action is said to be the means. For him who has ascended [to the summit of] Yoga, quiescence (*shama*) is said to be the means. (VI.3)

Shankara and Ramanuja, the two most prominent classical commentators on the *Gita*, interpreted the decisive term "quiescence" in the sense of "withdrawal from all action." However, this is clearly wrong. In the context of Krishna's integral doctrine, the word *shama* should be understood as indicating the kind of inner openness that is a precondition and the immediate result of the enlightenment experience. At that stage, the adept is indeed active without doing anything. Whatever action he or she performs is of the nature of a spontaneous manifestation of God's purpose or will.

One must guard against the precipitate conclusion that the adepts on that level are in any way possessed by some supranatural entity. There is no room for duality in their realization and activity. They have become the Whole, and therefore whatever they do on the empirical level is of necessity an expression of the Whole.

These masters, established in enlightenment, can no longer be perturbed by sorrow. They may still experience physical pain, but, lacking an egoic center, they do not make a mountain out of a mole hill. In other words, they transcend suffering, even though their body may be racked with pain, as was the case with Ramana Maharshi, who suffered from cancer toward the end of his life. Having reached the transcendental Continuum, the all-pervasive Being, they see all things in the same light.

By way of contrast, the practitioner who is still on the way, the *arurukshu*, relies on a certain code of conduct and a body of disciplines. The spiritual endeavor of such aspirants is a form of effort, which is associated with apparent progress and setbacks. Apart from their daily work, executed in the light of the ideal of inaction-in-action, they stand in need of specially set-aside hours of quiet contemplation during which they make an intensified effort to direct their mind toward the Divine.

According to the *Gita*, meditative absorption (dhyana) is the fervent orientation of one's whole being to the transcendental Reality. This self-offering can be compared to the affective prayer in Christian worship. Krishna is averse to any thought acrobatics or intricate psychotechnical practices. He favors a spontaneous, unforced approach, and his teaching is a true middle path. This can be seen, for instance, in the fact that he does not recommend breath control in the way it was propagated in later times, with excessive retention of the breath. Krishna's only instruction about the practice of pranayama is contained in a single stanza:

> Shutting out [all] external contacts and [fixing] the gaze between the eyebrows, making even the inflow and out-flow [of the life force] moving within the nostrils, [the yogin approaches liberation]. (V.27)

The God-man recommends that spiritual practitioners be circumspect and simple in everything. Krishna's message centers throughout on balance, and the word *sama*, meaning "equal" or "even," occurs in numerous compounds, such as *samatva* (balance) or *sama-darshana* ("vision of sameness"). The aspirants must avoid all extremes, within themselves and without. Only thus can they ultimately discover Krishna's "imperishable Yoga" and thereby transcend all duality.

As Krishna Prem, a Westerner who went to India to hear the divine song in his own heart, reminded us in his outstanding book on the *Gita*, Krishna's eternal wisdom is not a body of doctrines with which one could agree or disagree.[5] It is the Truth itself, which must be discovered in the lightning-flash of illumination.

Krishna's incarnation on Earth was simply meant to re-ignite the spiritual fire within his contemporaries, who had lost sight of the earlier sacred revelation. His song of instruction, available today in hundreds of versions around the world, still has the same purpose of rekindling the spiritual flame in human hearts. But to hear that song rightly, we must not get distracted by the inevitable archaism of his language and thoughts but look beyond to the eternal Mystery to which Krishna and a thousand other sages in India and elsewhere have pointed.

NOTES

1. Thus there is the *Uttara-Gita*, the *Ganesha-Gita*, and the *Uddhava-Gita*, to mentioned but a few.

2. This teaching is associated with the Hindu adept and theologian Ramanuja. See the pertinent remark by J.A.B. van Buitenen, *Ramanuja on the Bhagavadgita* (Delhi: Motilal Banarsidass, 1968), p. 39: "[Ramanuja] has completed the task which the poet of the Gita had begun, the reconciliation of thought and religion."

3. See *Bhagavad-Gita* V.2 and III.7.

4. S.N. Dasgupta, *A History of Indian Philosophy* (Cambridge: Cambridge University Press, 1965), vol. 2, p. 486.

5. See K. Prem, *The Yoga of the Bhagavat Gita* (London: Stuart & Watkins, 1969), pp. 30–31.

CHAPTER 27

LOVE, HUMAN AND DIVINE

SPIRITUAL ASCETICISM TEMPERED BY LOVE

The *Bhagavad-Gita* promotes an integral view of life, a fact that some interpreters have overlooked when trying to assign a fixed label to Krishna's teaching, identifying it as either *jnana-yoga*, *karma-yoga*, or *bhakti-yoga*. The truth is that the path outlined in the *Gita* integrates the cognitive and conative, as well as affective aspects of human nature. No human faculty is denied expression, but each is first harmonized and then put to use in the great quest for, and celebration of, the Divine.

Normally, our emotional life is fragmented into countless fleeting feelings of fear, attachment, repulsion, greed, anger, and so forth. For this reason, the program of mythic spirituality is geared to terminating all these emotions. But this is not the answer that Krishna proposes. He does not deny the affective side of our inner life, but instead advises us to transmute and then employ our refined feelings to reach spiritual perfection.

Specifically, the innumerable desires through which we tend to lose ourselves to insignificant external things have to be gathered into a single laserlike current of ardent devotion to the Supreme. This is what is meant by bhakti, the loving adherence to, and participation in, the Divine. Bhakti is the unqualified turning of one's whole being to the omnipresent Origin. In the words of philosopher and statesman Sarvepalli Radhakrishnan:

> Every drop of one's blood, every beat of one's heart, and every thought of one's brain are surrendered to God.[1]

The *Bhagavad-Gita* differentiates between two stages of bhakti. At the lower stage the dualism between the lover and the Beloved is not yet transcended, whereas at the higher stage there reigns perfect communion of love in eternal bliss and emancipation. In subsequent periods, the emotive element in Vaishnavism came to be greatly emphasized and was instrumental in the emergence of the so-called "way of devotion" (*bhakti-marga*). This grew into a cultural movement that covered many traditions and was immensely popular in both Northern and Southern India during the eighth to twelfth centuries A.D.

In the South, it was the high-flung devotional poetry of the twelve Alvars that inspired many generations of pious Vaishnavas. The Alvars are venerated as partial incarnations of God Vishnu. The songs of these poet-saints, who flourished in the eighth and ninth centuries A.D., express an ardent longing for the Divine in the form of Krishna.

Thus Tiruppan, of whom only a single poem has survived, rejoices:

> The blue-hued Lord,
> the cowherd boy and butter thief,
> has stolen my heart.
> O foremost of the Gods,
> Lord of Shriranga [temple],
> these blessed eyes of mine
> have gazed upon your beauteous form.
> May they never behold any other.

The saints Tirumangai and Namm composed between them half the Alvar poems gathered into the collection known as *Nalayira-Divya-Prabandham*, consisting of approximately four thousand hymns. Tirumangai, who lived in the eighth century, was a chieftain who abandoned his sybaritic ways in favor of a life of renunciation—all because of his love for Kumudavalli, a devout Vaishnava maiden. According to legend, the girl agreed to marry him on the condition that he provide a daily meal for 1008 Vaishnava devotees for an entire year. Tirumangai spent his entire fortune to meet the demand, and when he had run out of money, he became a Robin Hood, waylaying and robbing the wealthy to feed the poor.

On one occasion, he stripped a traveling brahmin and his wife of all their possessions but did not have the physical strength to carry away his loot. Suspecting that he was impeded by a magical spell, he demanded an explanation from the brahmin. The man remained silent, but Tirumangai heard with his inner ear the sacred mantra "Om, Obeisance to Narayana" (*om namo narayanaya*). He was so enchanted by this mantra that he grew more and more exuberant reciting it. Promptly the brahmin and his wife revealed their true identity as Lord Vishnu and his divine consort.

Tirumangai fell to his feet and on the spot was transformed. In due course, he married Kumudavalli but spent the rest of his life pilgrimaging from temple to temple, all the while composing and singing hymns of praise in honor of Vishnu's greatness.

The most revered Alvar is Namm, who is also known as Maran. He is said to have adopted a life of contemplation when still in his infancy. He emerged from his profound meditative state only at the age of sixteen. At that time, Madhurakavi went to the young saint and posed to him the following riddle: "When the small is born in the dead, what will it eat and where will it lie?" Namm opened his eyes, gazed at the visitor, and responded: "It will eat the dead and lie on it." Madhurakavi became Namm's first disciple.

Namm Alvar was not only a great b*hakta* but also a versatile and powerful poet. In one of his hymns, he sings:

The sandal paste he wears
is indeed my very heart.
The flower buds adorning him
are my words of praise.
My garland of praise
is indeed his silken cloth.
His gleaming jewels
are my humble folded hands.[2]

Thou art with me.
The flood of ecstasy as they touch
Overflows the sky
And I am drowned, sense and all.
Ah, but it is a dream, only a dream.
Thou art going
And the passion of yearning flares up again

And eats deep, deep into me.
No, no, life cannot bear it,
Thy going after the kine
May that die![3]

Here Namm assumes the role of a lovesick shepherdess (*gopi*)
longing for her beloved, Krishna, whose visits are too rare and
brief and merely cause her heartache. In some poems, Namm
speaks in touching ways as the mother of the shepherdess, inter-
ceding with the Lord on the maiden's behalf.

In the early ninth century lived the woman saint Andal. Like
Namm, she was absorbed in divine contemplation while still a
child. She knew that she would never marry a mere mortal, dedi-
cating her body and soul to Lord Vishnu. She constantly visualized
herself as the Lord's bride, and quite innocently used the garlands
at the local temple to decorate her body so that God Vishnu might
find her worthy of his attention.

When Peryalvar, the temple priest and the girl's adopted
father, discovered Andal's unpardonable transgression, he proceeded with the day's ritual without the use of the desecrated garland. That night, Vishnu appeared to Peryalvar in a dream, revealing to him that Andal was a blessed devotee and that her habit of
wearing the garland was pleasing to the Lord. Later, the priest told
the sixteen-year-old girl that God Vishnu had instructed him to
bring her into the inner sanctum of the temple in full bridal attire.
Legend has it that when the radiantly happy Andal stood before
Vishnu's stone statue, she was absorbed into it, becoming one with
her Beloved.

Two of Andal's lyrical compositions have been handed down
over the ages. The thirty verses of the *Tiruppavai* were and still are
very popular, whereas the *Nacciyar Tirumoli* is hardly known,
probably because its fourteen poems contain occasional erotic im-
agery that is not easy to reconcile with conventional piety. In one of
her hymns, Andal sings:

O rain clouds,
from whose bulk
lightning flashes forth,
tell the Lord of Venkata,

upon whose glorious body
reclines the Goddess Shri,
that I constantly yearn
for him to desire
the budding breasts
of my radiant body;
that he should visit
and hold me in his embrace.[4]

Andal expresses her great need for the Lord's love, praying
that he may enter her and consume her womanhood, as a gnat enters the woodapple and hollows it. She accuses her Beloved of tor-
turing her by his deliberate absence, and promises to be his slave
forever if only he would come to her.

The metaphor of slavery is common to the saintly bards of
South India. It is also shared by the Nayanars, the sixty-three mystical poets who worshipped the Divine in the form of Shiva rather
than Vishnu. Four of this group won special favor among the devout men and women of the South. Saint Appar, who lived in the
early seventh century, was a Jaina who had converted to Shaivism
after having been miraculously healed from a stomach complaint
at the Shiva temple of Virattanam.

Appar saw himself as the Lord's servant-slave (*dasa*), barely
worthy of singing Shiva's praise. In one of his much-loved songs,
he exclaims exuberantly:

I have seen them!
I have seen them!
I have seen the blessed feet of the Lord.
Those very feet that
I had never before seen,
I have now gazed upon.[5]

Another inveterate mystical songster and a contemporary of
Appar was Sambandar. His songs frequently extol in quite sensuous terms the beauty of Shiva's celestial spouse, Parvati. According to legend, it was none other than the Goddess who had given
Sambandar a cup of milk when he, as a young child, was waiting
one day for his father to emerge from the sacred waters of the

temple bath at Chidambara. Unlike Appar, who addressed Shiva
in most respectful terms befitting a servant, Sambandar regarded
himself as an intimate lover of God and Goddess.

An even more intimate, and for some ears even offensively familiar, style of approach to the Divine can be found in the poetry of
the eighth-century bard Sundarar, who was known for it as the
"insolent devotee." According to legend, Sundarar, as his name
suggests, was exceedingly handsome. In fact, the local ruler found
the boy's beauty so enchanting that he adopted him from his
brahmin parents. On his wedding day, the chieftain spent lavishly
on the preparations for the feast.

Just as Sundarar was about to be married, an old man stepped
forward and announced that the marriage could not proceed because the brahmin-born Sundarar was his slave. Somehow the old
man was able to procure documents to prove his claim, and so, to
everyone's astonishment, the village council ruled that Sundarar
had to go with him. The young man felt cheated out of the best day
of his life by what he perceived to be a complete madman. But he
followed in obedience to the judgement of theelders.

The wizened man walked faster and faster, and it was difficult
for Sundarar to keep step with him. Then his alleged master entered the temple of Vennai Nallur and vanished in the inner sanctum. It dawned on Sundarar that the old man was none other than
God Shiva himself. Then the Lord's voice reached his ears, demanding that henceforth Sundarar, the insolent devotee, should
worship him with song.

In the ninth century A.D., Manikkavachakar reached great fame
for his devotional hymns. When he was still a minister of King
Varaguna Pandya, he was sent on a mission to purchase the finest
horses he could find. Alas, Manikkavachakar, waylaid by God
Shiva himself, used the king's large sum of money to construct a
temple.

Shiva insisted that Manikkavachakar return to the royal court,
and promised that the horses would follow shortly. Shiva, in the
guise of a merchant, did indeed deliver the horses to King Varaguna. However, the following night they turned into jackals,
whereupon the hapless minister was promptly thrown into prison.
Shiva had to intervene again to free his new devotee.

Manikkavachakar's poems have stirred thousands of hearts. So have the hymns of the minstrels of the North, such as the Bauls of Bengal, who also proclaimed the path of devotion as the best and easiest way of gaining access to the Divine. Many of the Northern poetic creations expressing the ideal of bhakti-yoga revolve around the Krishna mythology developed in the *Bhagavata-Purana*. This massive ninth-to-tenth-century work has enjoyed immense popularity, surpassed only by the *Bhagavad-Gita* itself.

The *Bhagavata-Purana* served as the foundation not only for the later Vaishnava religious poetry but also for the great theological works of Ramanuja, Madhva, Vallabha, and Caitanya.

The devotionalism favored by these saintly preceptors stands in striking contrast with the long tradition of unemotional asceticism. At times, however, the devotional element of love (bhakti) and surrender (prapatti) was so exaggerated that it eclipsed both the Yoga of wisdom and the Yoga of action. The *Gita* translator W.D.P. Hill rightly commented:

> The *Gita* recognizes that no true religion should ignore emotion, and that no true emotion should isolate itself from the functions of reason and will; the balanced man must develop to its best every element that makes up the personality. But it was not long before emotionalists began to preach that ecstasy was all; sound study was ignored; the wild hysterical dance and the passionate repetition of the sacred name began to take the place of the more unexciting duties of the home and the simple service of mankind. The later *bhaktas* made the same mistake with *bhakti* that the earlier *jnanins* had made with *jnana*; isolation and over-emphasis ruined the very mode of approach they desired to exalt.[6]

Composed well over two millennia ago, the *Bhagavad-Gita* was still oblivious of the complicated theological and doctrinary reflections on bhakti that are so characteristic of later Vaishnavism. For Krishna, bhakti is the simple and direct alignment of the heart to God. He does not tear it from the context of an active life in the world according to the principles of dharma, nor does he separate it from the striving for enlightenment.

By seeing in everything the presence of the Divine and by

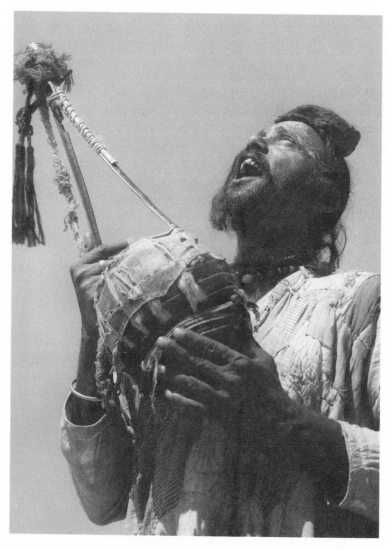

A Bengali bard of the Baul sect singing in praise of the Divine.
Photo by permission of Richard Lannoy.

casting off all mundane attachments, the aspirants of Krishna's integral spirituality are able to "detoxicate" daily life and hence no longer need take flight from it. With their mind immersed in the Divine, they are active in the world for the promotion of the welfare and ultimate liberation of all beings.

SELF-REALIZATION AND SUCCOR FOR HUMANITY

The social ideal of the *Gita* is epitomized in the Sanskrit term *loka-samgraha*, which literally means the "bringing together of the world." By becoming the "tool" of God, the yogin helps to sustain and articulate the harmony intrinsic in the universe. However, the ideal of loka-samgraha is neither ill-conceived altruism nor a cloaked plea for proselytism, because it is interwoven with the stringent spiritual demand to become one with the Divine.

In Krishna's ethics, Self-realization and participation in the affairs of the world are not antithetical. Rather, they are complementary poles of one and the same process of self-transcendence.

This was not accepted by the great adept and theologian Ramanuja, who lived in the eleventh century A.D. Ramanuja thought that all action is bound to spiritual ignorance. At the same time, however, he maintained that through karma-yoga, we can purify ourselves sufficiently to allow the dawning of discernment (jnana). Then, with the growth of our understanding, we become capable of devotion (bhakti) and thus receptive to God's grace. Ramanuja also felt that all work must be conducted as service to the Lord.

In the fifteenth century, an Assamese follower of Ramanuja by the name of Shankaradeva clearly upheld the ideal of social service, as borne out by the following traditional story. One day, Shankaradeva noted the absence of one of his pupils during one of their prayer meetings. He discovered that the missing disciple was attending a sick friend instead. When the other disciples expressed their disapproval, Shankaradeva reminded them that to serve a fellow human being is to serve the Divine.[7]

Not surprisingly, it is among the preachers of devotionalism that we find the most outspoken critics of the age-old institution of castes and other forms of inequality seemingly built into traditional Hinduism. Their ethical teachings represent crucial integral innovations, even though they were not always successful in permanently changing social attitudes and practices. Yet, undoubtedly, their courageous challenge of established mores has kept up the momentum of the integral consciousness, whose first stirrings are immortalized in the teachings of the *Bhagavad-Gita*.

NOTES

1. S. Radhakrishnan, *Indian Philosophy* (New York: Macmillan/London: Allen & Unwin, 1931), vol. 2, p. 705.

2. *Tiruvaymoli*, first decade, hymn 3, verse 2. Translated by V. Dehejia, *The Slaves of the Lord: The Path of the Tamil Saints* (New Delhi: Munshiram Manoharlal, 1988), p. 111.

3. Translated by A. Srinivasa Raghavan, *Nammalvar* (New Delhi: Motilal Banarsidass, 1975), p. 40.

4. Adopted from the translation by V. Dehejia, *Antal and Her Path of Love: Poems of a Woman Saint from South India* (New York: SUNY Press, 1990).

5. Adopted from the rendering by V. Dehejia, *The Slaves of the Lord: The Path of the Tamil Saints*, p. 35.

6. W.D.P. Hill, *The Bhagavadgita* (London: Oxford University Press, 1953), pp. 67–chapter 27 23068.

7. Yet, the same Shankaradeva, like his preceptor Ramanuja, denied women the privilege of joining his sect or studying the sacred tradition.

CHAPTER 28

LIBERATION IN THE EMBODIED STATE

THE MANY MANSIONS OF THE DIVINE

Transcendence of the mind in ecstasy leads to the abolition of the ordinary categories by which we apprehend the world. Space and time cease to exist in their well-known configuration, because the predictable boundary between subject and object is melted down. The resulting realization, however, is not invariably the same. This fact has been spelled out very clearly by Mircea Eliade, who commented:

> [It] is important to state that all expressions of the *coincidentia oppositorum* are not equivalent. We have observed on many occasions that by transcending the opposites one does not always attain the same mode of being. There is every possible difference, for instance, between spiritual androgynisation and the "confusion of the sexes" obtained by orgy; between spiritual regression to the formless and "spooky" and the recovery of "paradisaical" spontaneity and freedom.[1]

In regard to the higher ecstatic experiences, the threefold distinction proposed by the British historian of religion R.C. Zaehner presents a workable hypothesis. As mentioned in a previous chapter, he suggested that mystical transcendence can occur with reference to the Divine, the Self, or Nature. He based this tripartite model on the liberation teaching of the *Bhagavad-Gita*. It is of course based on an ontology that distinguishes between the Divine and the transcendental Self—a distinction that is not accepted by all schools. For instance, it would make no sense in the framework of Shankara's radical nondualism.

However, if we accept a theistic metaphysics, Zaehner's model is plausible enough. At any rate, we must accept that liberation is conceived differently in the various traditions. Whether these conceptual distinctions represent ultimate ontological differences is an unresolved issue. From the viewpoint of most of the spiritual traditions, their ideological disagreements are not merely doctrinal quibbling but actually are based on factual, experiential differences.

In other words, Ramanuja considers his form of liberation superior to the liberation taught by Shankara, because it is truer to the facts. Shankara, again, would argue with Ramanuja that the latter's notion of salvation is tainted and inadequate. The Hinayana Buddhists dismiss both their views as pure metaphysical speculation, whereas the Shunyavada school of later Buddhism only permits the "void."

Modern students of mysticism are divided into two broad camps. The first camp is made up of "perennialists" like William James, Aldous Huxley, Rudolf Otto, Mircea Eliade, W.T. Stace, and Huston Smith, who all maintain that mystical realization involves an unmediated contact with a transcendental reality, which is subsequently interpreted in various ways. The second camp comprises "constructivists" like Steven T. Katz, John Hick, and Peter Moore. This perspective was dominant in the 1980s, mainly through Katz's eloquent work.[2]

This articulate philosophical position has recently been challenged by a new model, which favors the existence of a "pure consciousness event" (PCE), because this is the repeated claim in the mystical traditions themselves.[3] As we have seen, ordinary consciousness is progressively deconstructed in the course of spiritual discipline, notably meditation. As a result, there arises a condition—ecstasy—similar to and often compared to the phenomenon of forgetfulness. The spiritual practitioner "forgets" to make the usual distinctions, especially the differentiation between himself or herself and the object of contemplation.

As we have also seen, the resultant condition is not one of unconsciousness but *pure awareness*. As Robert K.C. Forman, the main spokesman for the third camp, remarked:

> It is important to note that what is forgotten altogether in the PCE is expressly stated by many mystics to include the very concepts and teachings of the mystical traditions themselves. When Eckhart talks for example about *gelazen* (letting

go), he expressly includes all notions of God—and his own belief system—as part of that which must be given up; . . . In short, to temporarily forget everything includes forgetting even the very belief system which may have led to that forgetting.[4]

Forman is careful not to suggest that the experience of pure awareness is common to all spiritual traditions. Rather, in his view, we can expect to encounter this experience, or references to it, in those schools of thought that also operate with a "forgetting" method. Forman also believes that many philosophical models, or languages, may be employed to express what he calls a PCE.

Forman's approach to understanding mystical realization is by no means the final answer, but it is a promising beginning in our endeavor to think critically about this elusive subject. In isolating "pure awareness" as an ultimate feature of mystical realization, he has effectively bridged the gulf between perennialists and constructivists. However, pure awareness (*cit*) is often regarded as only one of several irreducible characteristics of mind-transcending ecstasy. Two other oft-mentioned characteristics are pure being (*sat*) and pure bliss (*ananda*). To this, some theistic schools add pure love (*bhakti* or *prema*).

LIBERATION AS LOVE-PARTICIPATION

The *Bhagavad-Gita* recognizes two types of liberation. These are really two stages of completeness in the salvific process. The lower stage is designated as *brahma-nirvana*, meaning "extinction in the world-ground"; the higher grade is the realization of love-participation in God's being.

The world-ground (brahman) is here the transcendental matrix of Nature, not the Absolute itself. Spiritual practitioners must beware of confusing ecstatic immersion into that world-ground with the ultimate goal of participating in the Divine. Once they have transcended all duality and achieved the state of transcendental oneness, they must next turn their liberated essential being toward the Divine. The brahma-nirvana is without love, which is the cherished fruit of the adept's awakening in God.

There is a striking parallel to this two-tier process in the teaching of the German mystic Meister Eckhart. In one of his German sermons, this great spiritual teacher said:

> [Wisdom] brings God into the soul and guides the soul to God.
> But it is unable to bring it right into God. Hence God does not
> accomplish his divine works in wisdom, because it is limited
> in the soul. However, [when the soul has approached God by
> means of such gnosis] then the uppermost power [of the soul]
> emerges—which is love—and breaks into God and leads the
> soul, together with wisdom and all its other powers, into God
> and unites it with God.[5]

A very similar mystical theology was put forward by the great
Vaishnava preceptor Ramanuja in the eleventh century A.D. He too
believed that wisdom alone is not a sufficient means of God-realization. Wisdom, he taught, can guide us only part of the way.
Then love must take over. In his *Veda-Artha-Samgraha* (126–127), a
popular compendium of Qualified Nondualism, Ramanuja outlines the steps by which such love is awakened in the heart. To
paraphrase his statement written in somewhat convoluted Sanskrit:

> The Supreme Person is realized by that spiritual practitio-
> ner who has accumulated extraordinary virtue, which eradi-
> cates all the sins piled up in his or her previous lives, and who
> faces inward seeking refuge at the lotus feet of the Supreme
> Person. Having acquired understanding about the nature of
> Reality through diligent study of the sacred lore with the help
> of qualified teachers, the student next learns to control the
> senses and the mind through the cultivation of asceticism, pu-
> rity, forgiveness, rectitude, mercy, nonharming, and discrimi-
> nation, as well as dedication to the performance of his or her
> allotted duties. He offers himself to the Supreme Person, and
> prompted by devotion, constantly praises, worships, remem-
> bers, and contemplates Him. Then the Supreme Person, over-
> flowing with compassion and delighted by the devotee's love,
> showers His grace upon the aspirant, which destroys his or
> her spiritual darkness. Consequently, the devotee's love grows
> into an uninterrupted, vivid, and immediate envisioning of
> the Supreme Person.

Ramanuja describes this all-absorbing, passionate devotion to God as *para-bhakti* or "supreme love," a gift of the Divine itself. The transcendental love that flows between God and the emancipated being is not of an emotional and even less of an intellectual nature. Perhaps one could describe it as inscrutable divine creativity: the Whole "communicating" with itself in the form of the human being, and vice versa. For Ramanuja and some of his followers, this paradoxical condition can only be realized after discarding the body.

This view represents a return to the mythic model of spirituality, which postulates a sharp gap between the Divine and the mundane, between above and below. A more integrated view had been arrived at fifteen hundred years earlier by the anonymous composer of the *Bhagavad-Gita*.

As opposed to Ramanuja's theology and the metaphysical systems of Classical Yoga and Classical Samkhya, the *Gita* teaches that the transcendental Reality is not antithetical to the world of phenomena and that liberation can be realized even during the embodied state. In fact, Lord Krishna's religious ethic clearly demands that every effort should be made to attain liberation in this very life.

This is the ideal of *jivan-mukti*, "living liberation," which is shared by those schools of thought that exhibit a distinct integral orientation. Sarvepalli Radhakrishnan captured the quintessence of this holistic concept very well when he remarked:

> Life eternal is not in the future of time. Every moment we stand on the frontier of time. Release is not a state after death but the supreme status of being in which the spirit knows itself to be superior to birth and death, unconditioned by its manifestations, able to assume forms at pleasure.[6]

Jivan-mukti is Being in Becoming, Eternity in temporality, the Unconfined in the confined. It is the abolition of all experience of duality and the attainment of the perfect wholeness that marks the all-comprising Reality. The yogin in whom this supreme integration has matured is said to be "established in gnosis" (*sthita-prajna*) or "established in gnostic vision" (*sthita-dhi*). He lives in the world but is no longer of it. In the words of the *Bhagavad-Gita* (II. 56–57):

He whose mind is unagitated in sorrow, who is devoid of longing during pleasurable [experiences], free from passion, fear, and anger—he is called a sage of steadied vision.

He who is unattached toward everything, who rejoices not at whatever good comes to him, nor hates whatever bad [experiences he may encounter]—his wisdom is well-established.

These verses, which emphasize the inner equilibrium of the liberated being, are complemented by the following stanzas that reveal some more positive characteristics, such as compassion, friendliness, dedication to the Supreme, and not shrinking from the world:

He who is without hatred for any being, who is friendly and compassionate . . . [that] yogin who is ever content, self-controlled, of firm resolve, with mind and wisdom-faculty offered up in Me, who is My devotee—he is dear to Me.

He from whom the world does not recoil and who does not recoil from the world and who is free from exultation, anger, fear, and agitation, is dear to Me.[7]

The moral virtues enjoined in these verses are further augmented in the *Yoga-Vasishtha*, the greatest classic on monistic Yoga based on the ethical activism of the *Gita*. As the Indian scholar S.N. Dasgupta has noted:

. . . here the saint, though absolutely unaffected by all pleasures and sufferings, by virtue and vice, is yet not absolutely cut off from us, for, though he has no interest in his own good, he can show enjoyment in the enjoyment of others and sympathy with the sufferings of others; he can be as gay as a child with children, and as serious as any philosopher when with philosophers or old men [. . .] He is absolutely unattached to anything, but is not cut off from society and can seemingly take part in everything without losing his mental balance in any way.[8]

To cite the *Yoga-Vasishtha* (V.77) itself:

He does not concern himself with the future, nor does he abide [exclusively] in the present, nor does he recollect [i.e., live in the memory of] the past, but he acts out of the whole. (7)

Sleeping, he is awake. Awake, he is like one asleep. Performing all [required] actions, he does nothing whatsoever inwardly. (8)

Interiorly always renouncing everything, without inner desires and performing externally what is to be done, he remains [completely] equable (*sama*). (9)

Remaining perfectly happy and experiencing enjoyment in all that is expected [of him], he performs all deeds, [ever] abandoning the misconception of doership. (11)

[He behaves] as a boy among boys; an elder among elders; a sage among sages; a youth among youths, [and as] a sympathizer among the well-conducted afflicted. (14)

He is wise, gracious, charming, suffused with his enlightenment, free from pressure (*kheda*) and distress, an affectionate friend. (16)

Neither by embarking on the performance of action nor by abstention, nor by [such concepts as] "bondage" or "liberation," "underworld" or "heaven" [can he be perturbed]. (19)

[For], when the objective world is perceived as the unitary [Being], then the mind fears neither bondage nor emancipation. (20)

This description has exercised a great influence on other native writers, especially some of the anonymous composers of later *Upanishads*. The *Yoga-Vasishtha*'s model of the liberated being also inspired the fourteenth-century sage Vidyaranya, who was prime minister of King Vijayanagara. In his *Jivan-Mukti-Viveka* (IV.1ff.), he states that liberation in life has five sacred purposes, namely to safeguard wisdom, to promote asceticism, to ensure the absence of discord, to bring about the cessation of suffering, and to produce supreme bliss.

It is evident from the traditional descriptions that the liberated sages, though they may engage in conventional activities, are far from being ordinary. They are masters of simplicity. Even though they may compose poems or music, write books, or assume the role of a teacher, priest, or family head, they are never caught up in their various roles but remain settled in the transcendental Self.

Their behavior may or may not be in consonance with traditional expectations, but whatever their actions may be, these great adepts transcend the common illusion of being an independent actor. Their behavior and their speech come from a deep still place. They are always authentic, never in conflict with themselves. These liberated men and women are, in a nutshell, whole human beings, fulfilling the great promise of our species Homo sapiens sapiens.

We can see in the *Yoga-Vasishtha*, which is perhaps the finest Sanskrit composition on Yoga, a more mature expression of the fundamental integral insight into the organic wholeness of Being-Becoming, first expressed in the *Bhagavad-Gita*. The last verse of the above-quoted passage from the *Yoga-Vasishtha* in particular prepares the way for the transition to the Tantric teachings, which took a further step in the direction of an integral spirituality. Unquestionably, the Tantric teachings inspired the author of the *Yoga-Vasishtha*, though his predilection for radical nondualism and illusionism did not permit him to fully adopt the metaphysics of polarity delineated in the Tantras. The revolutionary spirituality of Tantrism will be discussed in chapter 30, but first we must examine some of the antecedent integral features within the Buddhist tradition.

NOTES

1. M. Eliade, *The Two and the One* (London: Harvill Press, 1965), p. 123, fn. 1.

2. See S.T. Katz, ed., *Mysticism and Philosophical Analysis* (London: Sheldon Press, 1978).

3. See R.K.C. Forman, ed., *The Problem of Pure Consciousness: Mysticism and Philosophy* (Oxford: Oxford University Press, 1990).

4. *Ibid.*, pp. 38-39.

5. J. Quint, ed., *Meister Eckehart: Deutsche Predigten und Traktate* (Munich: Carl Hanser Verlag, 1955), p. 368. The quote is from sermon 45.

6. S. Radhakrishnan, *The Brahma Sutra: The Philosophy of Spiritual Life* (London: Allen & Unwin, 1960), p. 215.

7. *Bhagavad-Gita* XII.13a–15.

8. S.N. Dasgupta, *A History of Indian Philosophy* (Cambridge: Cambridge University Press, 1973), vol. 2, p. 247.

CHAPTER 29

INTEGRAL BREAKTHROUGHS IN MAHAYANA BUDDHISM

HINAYANA AND MAHAYANA

Just as the ascetic tradition within Hindu society had received a creative jolt through the integral teaching of the *Bhagavad-Gita*, so several centuries later the heterodox tradition of Buddhism underwent a comparable galvanization. The breakthrough to a more integral position in Buddhism occurred at the beginning of the Christian era when the Buddhist community split into Hinayana and Mahayana schools.

This schism was effectively prepared at the second Buddhist Council convened in 383 B.C., a hundred years after the Buddha's death. At that time, the *maha-sanghikas* or "followers of the great order" accused the *sthavira-vadins* or "elders" of pursuing a selfish goal in seeking merely their own liberation and showing no concern for all other beings in need of salvation. It was this catholic attitude that gradually led to the emergence of the many schools of Mahayana Buddhism.

Whatever these internal antagonisms in the ancient Buddhist community may have been, we must be careful not to regard them as exposing shortcomings in the original teaching of the Buddha. For as is evident from the Pali canon, the Buddha himself appears to have taken a far less extremist viewpoint than would appear from the attitudes of some of his followers. Nevertheless, this great division of the Buddhist *sangha* is an indisputable historical reality, and one which can only be understood in depth if it is interpreted as the dawning of a more integral awareness at the predominantly mythic horizon of older Buddhism.

The sovereign ideal of the Hinayana, or "little vehicle," is nirvana (Pali: *nibbana*), which literally means "not blowing" and is commonly translated as "extinction." It refers to the cessation of all typically human desires, notably the lust for life itself, whereupon all suffering is transcended. Nirvana is the opposite of samsara, the phenomenal world. As Roger J. Corless explained:

> Nirvana is the end of samsara. Samsara is reality as we know it. We experience ourselves as space-time beings with definite, demonstrable limits on our actions of body, speech, and mind. Nirvana, or liberation, is the disappearance of our reality. . . . If everything we know disappears, it is impossible to imagine what might take its place, for, as samsaric beings, we can only imagine the new things as something like the old things. Yet the end of the space-time universe is *without analogy* and even to call it a "new thing" is to miss the mark.[1]

However, this no-thing-ness of nirvana has not prevented generations of Buddhists from picturing it in certain ways. As the English Buddhist Bhikshu Sangharakshita noted, in Hinayana quarters, nirvana is typically conceived as "actually existing 'out there' with a real path leading up to it as though to the door of a house."[2]

The Hinayana monks hail nirvana as the highest possible aspiration a human being can have. In fact, they present it as a categorical imperative: We must exert ourselves to the utmost in order to terminate our experience of suffering. It was precisely this individualistic orientation of the Hinayana that provoked the criticism and reproach of the Mahayana followers, who were quick to point out that besides being incomplete and onesided, the fostering of thoughts of one's personal salvation runs counter to the Buddha's gospel:

> A sage of great insight thinks at once of his own liberation, of the liberation of others and of the liberation of the whole world.[3]

The revision of the Buddhist goal was not the only innovation that the Mahayana introduced. There were other dramatic developments occasioned by a profound general change of attitude, reflecting a more integral awareness. Bhikshu Sangharakshita summarized the most conspicuous features of this overall reevaluation thus:

The Hinayana being conservative and literal-minded, scholastic, one-sidedly negative in its conception of Nirvana and the Way, over-attached to the formal aspects of monasticism, and spiritually individualistic, the Mahayana, as a movement of reaction against the Hinayana, was naturally compelled to emphasize the importance of whatever qualities and characteristics were the exact opposite of these.[4]

The learned author singled out the following points of distinction, stating that the Mahayana

1. is more liberal-minded and progressive;

2. pays greater attention to the emotive aspect of human nature, favoring a more devotional attitude and betraying a deeper understanding of ritual worship;

3. is more positive in its conception of the goal and the path;

4. gives increased importance to a dedicated householder life, thereby bridging the gulf between lay Buddhists and the monastic order, without however denying the monastic ideal;

5. cultivates the altruistic component of Buddhism in preaching the *bodhisattva* ideal.

Whereas the older Buddhism was predominantly concerned with psychological realities, showing a conspicuous dislike for metaphysical speculations and epistemological facts, the Mahayana unmistakably rests on strong idealistic foundations.[5] The phenomenal world is compared to an apparition, and the reality of suffering—which preoccupied the Hinayana monks—is similarly taught to be illusory. There is only the absolute Void (*shunya*), understood as a self-existent continuum.

This monistic conception closely approaches the doctrine of brahman in Advaita Vedanta. In fact it is quite feasible that the nondualistic (*advaita*) strand of Hinduism was decisively inspired by Mahayana thought. The striking epistemological affinity between these two spiritual traditions is most eminently apparent in the teaching of Gaudapada, the father of philosophical nondualism and the teacher of Shankara's teacher. Of specific interest is his so-called "Yoga of noncontact" (*asparsha-yoga*), which is introduced in the *Mandukya-Karika* thus:

The Yoga of noncontact is difficult to be realized by all [ordinary] yogins. [These] yogins shrink back from it, imagining fear [where there is] no fear. (III.39)

All [ordinary] yogins depend on the restraint of consciousness for fearlessness, the destruction of sorrow, enlightenment, and imperishable peace. (III.40)

When consciousness is latent (*laya*),[6] it should be awakened; when distracted, it should be pacified again. [In the intermediary state] know [the mind to contain] desires [which again and again upset the mental equilibrium]. When [consciousness] is balanced out, it should not be disturbed again. (III.44)

[Consciousness] must not [be allowed to] bathe in the bliss [arising] from that [ecstatic experience] but should be detached [from it] through insight (*prajna*). When immobile and steadied, consciousness should be unified with effort. (III.45)

The fear that the ordinary yogins experience in facing the abyss of the ultimate Reality shows that they have not yet transcended the realm of duality, for where there is one only, *the* One, fear cannot arise.[7] The unillumined consciousness recoils in terror from the transcendental Singularity, as revealed in the Yoga of noncontact. The reason for this is that realization of that ultimate Being spells the end of the ego-identity, the finite personality. All the individual mind can see is the prospect of its own demise, and so it fearfully equates the Absolute with an unending vacuum, the absence of all that it holds dear.

There is also an important difference between the quasi-yogic exercise of rendering the mind insensate by forcing it into a state of oblivion, known as jada-samadhi in Sanskrit, and the genuine realization of the nondual Absolute. It is by means of the latter event that mind becomes Mind. States Gaudapada in perfect Mahayanic fashion:

This [phenomenal world] of duality, characterized by subject and object, is a mere quivering of consciousness (*citta-spandita*), wherefore Mind (*citta*) is declared to be devoid of objects, eternal and without contact. (IV.72)

Now, if the world has only an apparitional character and if not even nirvana can strictly be said to exist, as the Mahayana teachers insist, then both mental constructs—"phenomenal world" and "transcendental Reality"—are in a certain sense equivalent and interchangeable. Indeed, this is exactly what the Mahayana scriptures affirm. For instance, in Nagarjuna's *Madhyamika-Shastra* (XXV.19–20), we find this statement:

There is no distinction between samsara and nirvana; there is no distinction between nirvana and samsara. The realm of nirvana is also the realm of samsara. Between them is not the slightest distinction.

The Void is the sole Reality, which the unenlightened mind conveniently but misleadingly fragments into two compartments—phenomenal existence and absolute existence. This mental habit of creating oppositions out of everything is a distinct trait of unenlightenment. To highlight the utterly transconceptual nature of Reality, the later Buddhist philosophers introduced the term "Void" or "Voidness."

Far from stopping the conceptual mind, however, this *shunya* has given rise to its own heritage of definitions and interpretations, as well as misunderstandings. One of the best renditions of the Sanskrit term *shunya* was proposed by Lama Anagarika Govinda, who wisely explained it as "transparency."[8]

The equation of samsara with nirvana is not only a fascinating philosophical innovation, superseding the mythic "above-below" scheme, it also has an important practical consequence. For, if nirvana does not lie outside the boundaries of phenomenal existence, then there is no need to abandon mundane life in search of it. Every being is in essence already enlightened, or liberated.

Hence those who try to take flight from the impinging actualities of phenomenal existence evidently still believe in, and reinforce, the artificial dualism of the unenlightened mind. This argument is pivotal to the Mahayana criticism of the Hinayana branch of Buddhism, which endows nirvana almost with a spatial quality.

THE COMPASSIONATE BODHISATTVA

The mythic orientation of the Hinayana tradition is epitomized in the figure of the solitary enlightened being, or *pratyeka-buddha*, who has won liberation on his own but who, unlike Gautama the Buddha, keeps his gnosis to himself and is not in the least motivated to share it with others. The Buddhist texts compare these retiring beings to the rhinoceros, which also lives on its own.

The figure of the self-made *buddha* has served large sections of the Buddhist community as an overt or covert ideal. A strong reclusive—and what the later Mahayana Buddhists perceived to be egocentric—attitude is also present in the common understanding of the life of the *arahants*, or "worthies," who have won the path to liberation thanks to Gautama's teaching.

In the *Dhamma-Pada*, an early Buddhist work, the arahant is described as a true brahmin. The following verses are characteristic of the tenor of this Pali text whose language is reminiscent of the Hindu *Bhagavad-Gita*:

One who does not associate
with either householders or homeless [ascetics],
who has no [fixed] abode and requires but little—
that one I call a brahmin. (404)

One who does not oppose among opponents,
who is pacified among those who are armed,
who does not grasp among those who grasp—
that one I call a brahmin. (406)

In whom no craving is found
for this world or the next,
who is released and [entirely] without craving—
that one I call a brahmin. (410)

The homeless one who, having given up lust,
goes forth, here [in this world],
and in whom [even] the lust for existence is extinct—
that one I call a brahmin. (415)

He who, having abandoned the human yoke (*yoga*),
has [likewise] transcended the heavenly yoke,
who is released from all yokes—
that one I call a brahmin. (417)

He who, having abandoned pleasure and displeasure,
has become cool, independent of [external] support,
a hero overcoming the entire world—
that one I call a brahmin. (418)

In contrast to the arahants and pratyeka-buddhas of Hinayana, the followers of the Mahayana path defer their own liberation until such time as all other beings are liberated. This is the
celebrated bodhisattva ideal. The bodhisattva, which means literally "enlightenment being," is the initiate who undertakes the
spiritual journey to enlightenment as an act of compassion for all
beings. What exactly this great Mahayana ideal entails can be seen
from the bodhisattva vow:

I take upon myself the burden of [all] suffering, I am resolved
[to do so]. I will endure it . . . I do not turn back or despond.
And why? At all cost must I bear the burdens of all beings. In
that I do not follow my own inclinations. I have made the vow
to save all beings.[9]

The bodhisattvas strive for complete enlightenment (*samyak-
sambodhi*) and are not content with what they perceive to be the
merely partial enlightenment of the arahants. Their indispensable
prerequisites for attaining that lofty goal are, first, the accumulation of merit through unwavering devotion to the weal of all
beings and, second, the accumulation of gnosis (jnana) through the
systematic cultivation of meditative inwardness.

The path of the bodhisattva consists of ten successive stages,
which are traversed with the help of the six (or sometimes ten)
"perfections" (*paramita*), or accomplished virtues:

1. *dana* — unconditional generosity even at the price of
               one's own well-being

2. *shila* — flawless moral conduct

3. *kshanti* — unlimited patience

4. *virya* — untiring exertion

5. *dhyana* — meditative absorption at all times

6. *prajna* — wisdom

Upon the consummate practice of these virtues, a person becomes a transcendental bodhisattva or, as the texts say, a "great entity" (*maha-sattva*). After death, instead of entering the static nirvana, such beings continue to work for the spiritual upliftment of all creatures. Their particular condition is known as *apratishta-nirvana* or "dynamic extinction."

Understandably, in the course of time, these universal saviors have become objects of awe, inspiration, veneration, and worship. They are the embodiment of wisdom *and* compassion. One of these great beings is Amitabha, or Avalokiteshvara. In Mahayana mythotheology, his transcendental work is glorified as follows:

> In the infinite blue sky of absolute space, the Buddha Amitabha sits, poised in the perfect peace of Transcendental Meditation. . . . As he gazes down at the universe, he feels utterly helpless. Transcendental being though he is, he cannot help everyone. So intensely does he enter into the individual agony of every creature that his body cannot absorb or express the power of his emotion and it bursts into fragments. His head splits into eleven pieces, each of which forms another head, searching yet more intently for beings in need. . . . No being, however minute, goes unnoticed. . . . Although he feels the pains of every other being as if they were his own, yet is he inseparably immersed in the supreme bliss of Transcendental Realization and, though he works without ceasing out of his bottomless Compassion, he feels his work to be a joyous play.[10]

The all-compassionate Avalokiteshvara is one among many such transcendental beings who untiringly exert themselves for the good of all creation. The Mahayana scriptures are full of legends about them.

The bodhisattva's self-chosen ordeal for the sake of others is all the more remarkable when we recall the metaphysical starting-point of Mahayana Buddhism, namely the axiom that the world of phenomena is void. Here the term *shunya* stands not, as in older Buddhist schools, for the transience and irrelevance of all created things. Rather, it signifies their true nature, which is the great Void, the transparent Origin.

This idea was greatly elaborated in the Madhyamika school, also called Shunyavada. Its founder was Nagarjuna (A.D. 150), an accomplished yogin and dialectician. He systematized and vindicated the teachings found in the *Prajna-Paramita* literature, which first expounded the Mahayana philosophy.

THE PATH OF RAPID ENLIGHTENMENT

In the early post-Christian era, the Buddhist culture appears to have been split into three camps. First, there were the monks and nuns who, to the best of their abilities, lived according to the strict monastic rules and dedicated much of their time to the activities of the order. Many of them were engaged in studies of various kinds. The second camp consisted of renouncers who preferred a contemplative life over monastic duties, and they often chose to retire to the forests or mountains. The final camp was made up of the large number of lay followers who were neither avid students of the Buddhist canon nor gifted meditators. They often resorted to a devotional attitude toward the Buddha, the bodhisattvas or arahants, and ordinary monks and nuns, hoping to acquire merit by supporting the order or individual monks or simply by being respectful of them.

An important branch of the ramified Mahayana tradition of those days in which meditative practice was placed in the foreground was the Yogacara school of Asanga (c. 350 A.D.). Its theoretical superstructure was supplied by the Vijnanavada of Vasubandhu, a brother of Asanga.

According to Vasubandhu, the ultimate Reality is pure Cognition (*vijnapti-matra*), which is solely responsible for the creation or, rather, imagination of the world of phenomena. Everything is mere ideation (*vikalpa*). Nothing is external to Mind. All that is required to realize this essential nondual Mind is the reversal (*paravritti*) of the ideation process. This is accomplished by means of yogic internalization, which deconstructs the habits of the ordinary consciousness.

The intense practical orientation of the Yogacara school culminated in the Chinese Ch'an school, which was founded by the Indian monk Bodhidharma early in the sixth century A.D. and flourished between the eighth and thirteenth centuries. It reached the island of Japan at about A.D. 1200, where it came to be known as Zen.

This school of thought decries all intellectualism and also dodges the devotionalism prevalent in some branches of Mahayana Buddhism. It insists that all traditional views and dogmas, in fact any concept, must be thrown overboard so that the spontaneous wu experience, or what in Japanese is called *satori*, can occur.

In order to confound the conceptual mind, the Zen masters work with paradox, as best exemplified in the "riddles" (*koan*) posed to students. These riddles are intellectually unsolvable. "What is the sound of one hand clapping?" What indeed? This approach amounts to a jujitsu attack, using the mind's momentum to defeat itself. This is quite different from the kind of forceful confinement of the mind characteristic of the mythic traditions. Rather, Zen in many ways represents an integral orientation.

This fact is also evident in its central spiritual realization, satori, which must not be equated with the yogic samadhi. The latter ecstatic state typically presupposes the suspension of sensory awareness and extreme inwardness of experience. It is the fruit of the mythic process of withdrawal from the outer world and complete concentration upon the inner reality.

Satori, however, is not necessarily preceded by such abstraction and self-encapsulation. On the contrary, the Zen practitioners, who understand that the phenomenal world is in truth the ever-present Reality, see no need for cutting themselves off from anything. This is reflected in their meditative practice of simply remaining mindful of all events even as they arise on the screen of consciousness. The integral path of Zen approaches realization from the waking consciousness. Satori can happen in any circumstance whatsoever—after sitting years in front of a blank wall, as did Bodhidharma, or while taking a bath, as was the case with Bhadrapala.

Hence D.T. Suzuki was able to claim that Zen is not mysticism, as ordinarily understood. As this venerable Zen teacher put it:

> Zen does not teach absorption, identification, or union, for all these ideas are derived from a dualistic conception of life and the world. In Zen there is a wholeness of things, which refuses to be analysed or separated into antitheses of all kinds.[11]

According to one of the countless Zen anecdotes, a Confucian scholar once visited a Zen master. He wanted to know what the ultimate secret of Zen was, and the master asked the scholar to join him on a walk along a mountain path. Passing by a blooming wild laurel tree, the master asked: "Do you smell that fragrance?" The scholar responded: "I do." The Zen master concluded the conversation saying: "Then I have hidden nothing from you."[12]

NOTES

1. R.J. Corless, *The Vision of Buddhism: The Space Under the Tree* (New York: Paragon House, 1989), p. 280.

2. Bhikshu Sangharakshita, *The Three Jewels* (London: Rider, 1967), p. 143.

3. *Anguttara-Nikaya* IV.186.4.

4. Bhikshu Sangharakshita, *A Survey of Buddhism* (Bangalore: Indian Institute of World Culture, 1966), p. 250.

5. H.V. Guenther has objected to the use of "idealism" in regard to Buddhism and even Western philosophy, suggesting the term "mentalism" instead. However, even his proposed alternative is barely adequate. Since the present book is not a philosophical treatise but written for the lay reader, I have retained "idealism" and "idealistic" throughout. See H.V. Guenther, *Buddhist Philosophy in Theory and Practice* (Harmondsworth, England: Pelican Books, 1972), p. 90.

6. The term *laya* refers to a peculiar ecstatic condition, known as *laya-samadhi*, in which all conscious activity is suspended. The yogin merges with the world-ground without, however, attaining to Being-Awareness. See *Yoga-Sutra* I.19 and the *Yoga-Bhashya* thereon.

7. When speaking of (ordinary) yogins, Gaudapada most likely has in mind the followers of Classical Yoga.

8. See A. Govinda, *Creative Meditation and Multi-Dimensional Consciousness* (Wheaton, IL: Theosophical Publishing House, 1976), p. 51. In his earlier works, Govinda translated *shunya* as "emptiness," and his switching to "transparency" was probably due to the influence of Jean Gebser. Roger Corless in his fine work *The Vision of Buddhism* independently proposed the same rendering.

9. *Shiksha-Samuccaya* XVI. This extract is from P. L. Vaidya's edition of the Sanskrit text (p. 148).

10. A. Kennedy, *The Buddhist Vision: An Introduction to the Theory and Practice of Modern Buddhism* (York Beach, ME: Weiser, 1987), pp. 189–190.

11. D.T. Suzuki, *Studies in Zen* (New York: Delta Books, 1955), p. 81.

12. Told by D.T. Suzuki, *Studies in Zen*, p. 199.

CHAPTER 30

THE TANTRIC REVOLUTION

THE EMERGENCE OF TANTRISM

The integrative teachings arising within Hinduism and Buddhism created a viable basis for a pan-Indian synthesis. This presented itself in the form of Tantrism. It seems that Tantrism first gained a foothold in the Mahayana Buddhist community and shortly thereafter also penetrated the Vedic or Hindu tradition.

Broadly speaking, Tantrism rounded off the protracted process of amalgamation that took place between Brahmanism and popular traditions. Indeed, the Tantric synthesis was even more comprehensive inasmuch as it also assimilated non-Indian cultural elements from adjacent countries such as Assam and Tibet.

Something of the expansiveness of Tantrism is unwittingly captured in the Sanskrit word *tantra* itself, which is derived from the verbal root *tan* meaning "to expand" or "to continue." According to an occult definition, tantra is "that which expands knowledge." The knowledge intended here, however, is not factual information but gnosis. Tantrism is a means of acquiring direct knowledge of the oneness of all existence.

The historical circumstances surrounding the emergence of Tantrism are still poorly understood. The earliest Tantric writings, called *Tantras* and *Agamas*, date back to the fifth century A.D. One of the oldest extant Tantric works is the *Guhya-Samaja* ("Secret Assembly"), a Buddhist text. By comparison, the earliest available Hindu *Tantras* such as the *Mahanirvana-Tantra* belong to the seventh century. Tantrism soon became what historian of religion Mircea Eliade called a vogue among philosophers, theologians, and spiritual practitioners. As he noted, in a comparatively short time all branches of Indian culture came under the influence of Tantrism.[1]

In the seventh century, Tantrism found its way into Tibet

where it grew into the distinct tradition of Vajrayana Buddhism, the "Diamond Vehicle." The term *vajra* ("diamond" or "thunderbolt") refers here to the ultimate Reality, which is indestructible. While Hindu Tantrism had to go underground during the British Raj, Buddhist Tantrism was able to thrive in Tibet until the Chinese invasion, and today many of its exponents live in Western countries. They are the last link in a very old spiritual tradition.

THE NATURE OF TANTRISM

Tantrism is, strictly speaking, not a philosophy or religion. Even less is it "a literary elaboration of the Stupa-worship of the laymen."[2] Rather, we must regard it as a full-fledged lifestyle, with its own distinct attitudes, values, and practices. For centuries it was a sweeping cultural movement, somewhat like European Romanticism, though more profound and complex as well as long-lived. Tantrism sees itself as authentically Buddhist or Hindu. Its revolutionary teachings are simply presented as adaptations to the changing conditions in the world.

The contribution of Tantrism to philosophy is negligible, and its uniqueness lies in the practical sphere, or what is called *sadhana*. It is this practical emphasis that prompted the noted Buddhist scholar Herbert V. Guenther to remark that "it is in Tantrism that Buddhism finds its efflorescence and constant rejuvenation."[3]

In the realm of philosophical ideas there is no break between Tantrism and the immediately preceding traditions. Buddhist Tantrism rests in the main on the foundations of the Madhyamika school of the Mahayana tradition, while its Hindu counterpart is solidly based on those of the nondualist school of Advaita Vedanta. Agehananda Bharati, Vedanta monk and American professor of anthropology, has made a special study of both Tantric movements. He elucidated the relationship between them as follows:

> There is decidedly such a thing as a common Hindu and Buddhist tantric ideology, and I believe that the real difference between tantric and non-tantric traditions is methodological: tantra is psycho-experimental interpretation of non-tantric lore. As such, it is more value-free than non-tantric traditions;

moralizing and other be-good doctrines are set aside to a far greater extent in tantrism than in other doctrine. By "psycho-experimental" I mean "given to experimenting with one's own mind," not in the manner of the speculative philosopher or the poet, but rather in the fashion of a would-be psychoanalyst who is himself being analysed by some senior man in the trade.[4]

In other words, Tantrism is essentially Yoga. Its basic temper is antispeculative and is often combined with a marked antiascetic attitude. The key-term is balanced practice. Lama Anagarika Govinda phrased this in the following way:

The Tantras brought religious experience from the abstract regions of the speculating intellect down to earth, and clothed it with flesh and blood; not, however, with the intention of secularizing it, but to realize it: to make religious experience an active force.[5]

THE PLURALISTIC APPROACH OF TANTRISM

The intensely practical approach of Tantrism has favored the inclusion of any conceivable method, even such methods as would be unthinkable within the circumference of mythic spirituality. Consequently, we find in the Tantras a veritable miscellany of practices, some of which represent the highest expression of spirituality while others belong to the magical realm.

The theoretical justification for this liberal orientation is found in the doctrine of the world ages (*yuga*). Tantrism professes to be the new message for the so-called *kali-yuga*, or dark age, when wickedness has reached its zenith and humanity has by and large become incapable of realizing the Self, or God, through the older techniques and means. These methods are said to have lost their efficacy. As the *Mahanirvana-Tantra* (II.20) states:

There is no other path to liberation and happiness in this life or in the next than the one revealed in the Tantras.

In this unwholesome age, which is traditionally thought to have commenced with Lord Krishna's death in 3006 B.C., all tricks, ploys, and devices are permissible in order to reach the pure Source, and everything that is mere theory, or book learning, can safely be cast aside.

The radical tolerance of Tantrism is both its strength and its weakness. On one hand, it was able to attract countless men and women who would otherwise never have tasted spiritual life; on the other hand, it has suffered from a persistent vulgarization and corruption of its lofty ideals.

The Tantric path allows for the personal psychological idiosyncrasies of initiates. For some it will only be possible to cultivate inwardness through external ritual, whereas others might find it more profitable to adopt the method of formless absorption. For instance, to those who are specially suited for spiritual life, the *Mahanirvana-Tantra* (II.12ff.) recommends the meditative recitation of the *brahma-mantra: om sac-cid-ekam brahma*, "*om*—the One Reality-Awareness, the Absolute." By this simple means, qualified practitioners are said to swiftly discover their true identity, as the Absolute.

Except for the fact that it has to be imparted by a propitious teacher to be successful, this practice is not connected with any other regulations. However, the *Mahanirvana-Tantra* (III.31) makes it clear that only those who succeed in developing what is called the mantra consciousness will benefit from this technique. Unless this change in consciousness is achieved, even a million repetitions of this sacred formula will be futile.

Mantra recitation is one of the most basic but vitally important instruments of the Tantric path. Other prominent means are the practice of *mudras, yantras*, and breath control, all of which promote the central practice of meditative visualization (dhyana). These aids are generally employed conjointly in a very complex ritual, which is at the core of Tantrism.

Of these implements, which utilize respectively sound, movement, and vision, mantra is an integral part of almost all Tantric approaches. According to an estimation by Agehananda Bharati, who tabulated twenty-five Hindu and ten Buddhist Tantras, about sixty percent of their subject matter is on mantras. What then is a mantra? Bharati supplied the following formal definition:

A mantra is a quasi-morpheme or a series of quasi-morphemes, or a series of mixed genuine and quasi-morphemes
arranged in conventional patterns, based on codified esoteric
traditions, and passed on from one preceptor to one disciple in
the course of a prescribed initiation ritual.[6]

This is a purely formal definition and hence says nothing
about the function of a mantra. It can have either of three purposes,
namely propitiation, acquisition, or identification. The first two
evince the magical origin of mantras: the warding off of illness or
evil influences and the acquisition of occult powers, as already
seen in the ancient *Atharva-Veda*.

The essential spiritual function of such sacred sounds is that of
identifying with the reality underlying a given mantra. On the
highest level, this means a complete merging with the Absolute.
As the famous Vedic mantra has it: *aham brahma asmi*, "I am the
Absolute."

As already indicated, in addition to mantras, Tantrism em-
ploys certain symbolic hand gestures called mudras ("seals"),
which derive from Buddhist iconography.[7] They accompany the
ritual acts and are the expression of a definite inner mood, consciously produced to enhance the process of introspection and
meditative introversion.

The third element that needs to be mentioned is the *yantra*
("instrument"). This is a geometrical figure drawn on specially
consecrated metal, cloth, or other substances, or simply into the
sand. Some yantras are also three-dimensional structures. The
symbolism of this device is rather intricate and becomes fully intelligible only in meditation when the yantra is activated.

Fundamentally, it is a representation of the universe in its multiple stratification. The Italian scholar Guiseppi Tucci, who has devoted an entire book to this intriguing subject, wrote about the
Buddhist *mandala* (which is a pictographic variant of the simpler
yantra) as follows:

It is, above all, a map of the cosmos. It is the whole universe in its essential plan, in its process of emanation and of
reabsorption. The universe not only in its inert spatial ex-
panse, but as temporal revolution and both as a vital process

which develops from an essential Principle and rotates round a central axis, Mount Sumeru, the axis of the world on which the sky rests and which sinks its roots into the mysterious substratum.[8]

But the yantra or mandala is not merely a cosmogram but a psychocosmogram, because the pattern of the objective reality coincides with that of the experiencing subject. Furthermore, the process of evolution and involution is repeated within the circle of the individual being, for microcosm and macrocosm share the same fundamental structure. Thus by meditatively entering the mandala, which is a simplified image of the universe, the adept gets in touch with the universe itself and with the deep structures of his or her own body-mind.

The crux of advanced Tantric practice is meditative absorption, which is mostly taught as visualization. Tantric visualization is extremely complex and is built up according to strict formulas. Its content is as a rule one of the many iconographic types representing enlightened entities and their corresponding levels of being.

The immediate purpose of this visualization is to achieve perfect identification with the vividly imagined deity or supramundane being. The next step is to gradually dissolve this internal, living image and through this process of dissolution enter the great Void. In other words, adepts first mentally create a prop on which to fix their attention, then merge with it in ecstatic identification, and finally erase it together with their own empirical identity.

This process—known as "Deity Yoga"—is like painting a lifelike image of oneself on canvas, transferring one's entire consciousness into it, only to erase the painting and with it one's own sense of individual being. Of course, there is a precious compensation for the loss of self-sense: the recovery of the all-pervasive Being beyond all possible qualification.

Tantrism also knows a formless method in which visualization plays no role. However, it appears that the path of form is thought to have one great advantage, namely that of producing an immense amount of psychic energy which, when properly utilized, can catapult the practitioner more safely toward the desired goal.

In Tibetan Tantrism the famous school of Naropa distinguishes six branches of the path of form:

1. Yoga of the inner fire (*gtum-mo*)[9]
2. Yoga of the illusory body (*sgyu-lus*)
3. Yoga of the dream state (*rmi-lam*)
4. Yoga of the clear light (*hod-gsal*)
5. Yoga of the intermediate state (*bar-do*)
6. Yoga of consciousness transference (*hpho-ba*)

These methods provide practitioners with a far more reliable map of the psychic landscape than is the case with the formless path. Nevertheless, the ultimate goal in both cases is the same realization of the Whole (*purna*) through which the world becomes as transparent as a crystal.

The same tolerant attitude that Tantrism shows in its practical sphere is also retained in regard to social relationships. Its practitioners (*tantrika*) discard in principle the rigid caste distinctions perpetuated in the orthodox brahmin-dominated community. However, in the case of Hindu Tantrism the abolition of caste is valid only during the actual performance of the Tantric rites.

The inner progress of practitioners is reflected in their progressive extrication from profane life. In accordance with the social ideal of Hinduism, the Hindu tantrikas begin their spiritual career as householders and later become renunciate householders. Finally, they enter the mendicant stage. The *Kula-Arnava-Tantra* mentions seven stages of initiation: *veda-acara* (Vedic approach), *vaishnava-acara* (approach of Vishnu worshippers), *shaiva-acara* (approach of Shiva worshippers), *dakshina-acara* (right-hand approach), *vama-acara* (left-hand approach), *siddhanta-acara* (approach in keeping with the complete doctrine), and lastly *kaula-acara* (approach of the Kaula adepts).

The first four levels belong to the path of worldly activity (*pravritti-marga*) and the last three to the path of cessation (*nivritti-marga*). These represent degrees of spiritual maturity rather than fixed successive layers of a preordained course.

SPIRITUAL EROTICISM

The crucial moment of the Tantric sadhana is the practitioner's entrance into the left-hand approach. Here the notorious panca-tattva ritual takes place. Another name for it is *panca-makara*, which refers to the five components of this ceremony which all begin with the letter *m*:

1. *madya* — wine
2. *mamsa* — meat
3. *matsya* — fish
4. *mudra* — parched grain
5. *maithuna* — sexual concourse

In the right-hand path, these are understood metaphorically, but in the left-hand approach they are taken literally. The first four ingredients are intended to act as stimulants, whereas the fifth, sexual congregation, is the climax of the ritual. The participants, all duly initiated, are seated in a circle, with the female participants to the left of the male practitioners. For the time of the ceremony both are regarded as hypostases of God and Goddess.

This ceremony is far from being a licentious adventure. Rather, it is a protracted ritual that demands utmost concentration and considerable self-control. The sexual union is not for experiencing physical pleasure, but for realizing that transcendental unity in which the masculine and the feminine cosmic principles are in eternal blissful congress. In other words, the goal of this infamous Tantric ceremony is *maha-sukha*, or transcendental delight.

In Buddhist Tantrism, which on this point is faithful to its ascetic-mythic provenance, the practitioner must under all circumstances avoid seminal emission. By contrast, in some schools of Hindu Tantrism, emission is the rule.[10] This practice is connected with the age-old Vedic idea of sacrifice (*yajna*). In offering up their life substance, semen, the male practitioners symbolically reenact the original sacrifice of the Creator in bringing forth the universe. However, most Tantric practitioners—Hindu and Buddhist alike—seek to preserve the semen.

Ritual coition is a highly symbolic act. It embodies the union of the masculine and feminine aspects of the primal Reality, which is naturally polarized in the human being. The conscious conduction of the feminine kinetic energy (*shakti*) to the masculine static energy (called *shiva* in the Hindu Tantras) is at the core of all Tantric discipline. Only through this process of reversal can the original state of undivided integration (*yuga-naddha*) be recovered.

This energy work is known as *kundalini-yoga*, which involves the awakening of the dormant energy at the base of the spine and its guidance to the psychospiritual center at the crown of the head. This yogic procedure will be described in more detail in the next chapter.

CELEBRATION OF THE FEMININE PRINCIPLE

Tantrism has led to a most remarkable reappraisal of the feminine element. In the pre-Tantric period, the female represented the very embodiment of evil and was denigrated as an obstacle on the spiritual path. The *Laghu-Yoga-Vasishtha* (I.2.95) contains a vivid reminder of this repressive attitude:

> Women are fuel to the fire of hell. [Apparently] lovely, they are [really] disastrous.

Contrast this with the Tantric approach, as for instance expressed in the *Mahanirvana-Tantra* (X.80a), where God Shiva addresses his divine spouse thus:

> Every woman is your effigy. You reside concealed in the forms of all women in this world.

In the immediately following line, one of the most horrible practices of the Hindus is condemned, namely the customary immolation of widows:

> That woman who, out of foolishness, ascends the funeral pyre of her husband, goes to hell.

In the *Prajna-Upaya-Vinishcaya-Siddhi* (V.22–23), we find the following statement:

> The Prajnaparamita must be adored everywhere by those who strive for liberation. Pure, she abides in the realm beyond this

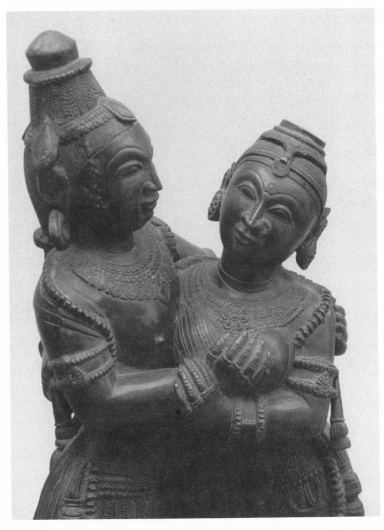

Statue of Krishna and Radha in loving embrace.
By courtesy of Open Secrets Bookstore, San Rafael, California.

empirical world. In this empirical world, she has assumed the form of [every] woman. In the disguise of woman, she is everywhere present . . .[11]

In Tantrism, woman is raised to the status of the incarnation of the divine Female. It would be misleading to see in this merely a revival of the indigenous Mother Goddess cult, which appears to have been prevalent already at the time of the Indus civilization. Tantric metaphysics is based on a clear understanding of the complementary polarity of male and female in the human psyche. And this is intimately connected with the Tantric key notion that phenomenal existence and transcendental Reality, samsara and nirvana, are not opposites but polar aspects of the Whole.

Their essential identity is realized when the human consciousness is cleansed of all misconceptions. Then both the flight from the world and the search for transcendence become meaningless; the mind no longer conceives of a path and a goal, but rests fulfilled in the all-pervasive Original Mind.

In the illuminating words of Lama Govinda:

By becoming conscious of the inner direction and relationship of our transient life, we discover the eternity in time, immortality in transiency,—and thus we transform the fleeting shapes of phenomena into timeless symbols of reality.

Liberation is not escapism, but consists in the conscious transformation of the elements that constitute our world and our existence. This is the great secret of the Tantras. . . . It is an act of resurrection, in which the ultimate transformation takes place and in which all causes come to rest in the light of perfect understanding and in the realization of *sunyata*, in which all things become transparent and all that has been experienced, whether in you or in suffering, enters into a state of transfiguration.[12]

THE WISDOM OF SPONTANEITY

In its latitudinarian approach, Tantrism comprises ritualistic schools as well as a freewheeling movement rejecting all ritual and doctrine. The latter is known as Sahajayana, or "Vehicle of Spontaneity," which straddled the great traditions of Buddhism,

Hinduism, and Jainism. The Sanskrit word *sahaja* means literally "together born (*ja*)," "coterminous" or "coessential." It is most commonly translated as "spontaneous/spontaneity," "natural," or "innate."

What it refers to is the fact that Reality is not separate from our ordinary world of experience. It is not a purely transcendental condition which has nothing to do with the empirical reality. Rather, there is only one Reality, which appears to the unenlightened mind as split into samsara and nirvana. For the enlightened being, however, the world is one.

From this radical perspective, there is no bondage to be suffered or liberation to be gained. There is no goal and no tortuous path of realization. The singleness of Reality is self-evident, and must simply become so obvious to the spiritual aspirant that all consciousness of duality is instantly abolished. The Buddhist adept Sarahapada, who lived in the eighth century A.D., compared the unenlightened individual to a fool who squints and takes the double image of a lamp for the lamp itself, or who looks in a mirror and mistakes the reflection of his face for the face itself, or who takes copper for gold, and colored glass for emerald.

Sahaja refers both to the naturalness of the innate Reality and the spontaneous way in which it can be realized. In view of this, the Sahajayana adepts presented their approach as the easiest road to liberation. For, as they argued, what could in principle be more natural than to simply recollect one's true nature? In practice, of course, this remembering of our true identity is the most difficult task confronting spiritual seekers, because their very search prevents them from seeing the truth.

Spiritual aspirants tend to make a path out of everything. They use rituals, mantras, yantras, self-castigation, sexual abstinence, and a hundred other means to force their way to the seemingly distant goal of liberation. Before they know it, the means have become goals in themselves. Hence in their popular poems, the adepts of the Sahajayana have poked fun at the typical aspirants who cling to the formalities of religious life, just as they have ridiculed scholarship.

These great adepts saw no need for pilgrimages, solitary dwelling in remote hermitages, endless recitation of magical formulas, daily bathing in the sacred rivers, or walking about naked clothed only in ashes. For them, all this was so much superstitious behavior. In the immortal words of Sarahapada:

> There's nothing to be negated, nothing to be Affirmed or grasped; for It can never be conceived. By the fragmentations of the intellect are the deluded Fettered; undivided and pure remains spontaneity.[13]

NOTES

1. See M. Eliade, *Yoga: Immortality and Freedom* (Princeton, NJ: Princeton University Press, 1973), p. 200.

2. E. Conze, *Buddhist Thought in India* (London: Allen & Unwin, 1962), p. 32, fn.

3. H.V. Guenther, "The Origin and Spirit of Vajrayana," *Stepping Stones*, No. 2, (May 1951), p. 4.

4. A. Bharati, *The Tantric Tradition* (London: Rider, 1965), p. 20.

5. Lama A. Govinda, *Foundations of Tibetan Mysticism* (London: Rider, 1972), p. 104.

6. A. Bharati, *The Tantric Tradition*, p. 111.

7. The term mudra ("seal") is used to signify a variety of things. In the Buddhist tradition it denotes the female partner in the sexual ritual. In Hindu Tantrism it stands for parched grain, one of the ingredients of the ill-famed *panca-tattva* rite of the left-hand path. In Hatha-Yoga it signifies certain bodily postures similar to the asanas. Lastly, in Buddhist Tantrism it is also used in the sense of "symbol," as in *karma-mudra*, *samaya-mudra*, *dharma-mudra*, and *maha-mudra*, which respectively refer to the female partner, the conventional meditative object, the realization of the Absolute, and the innate joy as the ultimate goal.

8. G. Tucci, *The Theory and Practice of the Mandala* (London: Rider, 1969), p. 23.

9. This word and the immediately following terms are in Tibetan.

10. Agehananda Bharati's claim that ritual ejaculation is characteristic of Hindu Tantrism in general is wrong.

11. This rendering is adopted from the translation by H.V. Guenther, *Yuganaddha—The Tantric View of Life* (Varanasi: Chowkhamba Sanskrit

Series Office, 1969), p. 83. The Prajnaparamita is here a personification of ultimate wisdom in the form of the great Goddess, rather like Sophia for the Gnostics.

12. A. Govinda, "The Two Aspects of Reality," *Main Currents in Modern Thought*, vol. 28, no. 4 (New Rochelle, 1972), pp. 129–130.

13. H.V. Guenther, *The Royal Song of Saraha: A Study in the History of Buddhist Thought* (Berkeley: Shambhala, 1973), p. 70. This is stanza 35 of Saraha's royal *doha*.

CHAPTER 31

THE SECRET TEACHING OF THE INDESTRUCTIBLE BODY

THE NEW VIEW OF THE BODY

The great adepts of Tantrism preached that the physical universe is spiritual in its essence. This reappraisal of bodily existence reached its climax in the endeavor to immortalize the human body in the schools of kaya-sadhana, or "body cultivation," especially Hatha-Yoga.

As we have seen, the ascetical traditions of mythic spirituality were at odds with the finite world and plotted the quickest way out of it. They typically viewed the body as the principal source of defilement, obscuring our innate freedom and bliss. This stereotype is reiterated in countless Hindu, Buddhist, and Jaina scriptures. One of the most dramatic denigrations of the human body can be found in the *Maitrayaniya-Upanishad* (I.3):

> Venerable one, in this ill-smelling, insubstantial body [which is nothing but] a conglomerate of bones, skin, sinews, muscles, marrow, flesh, semen, blood, mucus, tears, rheum, feces, urine, wind, bile, and phlegm—what good is the enjoyment of desires? In this body, which is afflicted with desire, anger, greed, delusion, fear, despondency, envy, separation from the desirable, union with the undesirable, hunger, thirst, senility, death, disease, sorrow, and the like—what good is the enjoyment of desires?

Many centuries later, the same negative view was expressed, for example, in the *Agni-Purana* (51.15–16):

> An ascetic regards his body at best as an inflated bladder of skin, surrounded by muscles, sinews and flesh, filled with ill-smelling urine, feces and dirt, a dwelling place of illness and suffering and an easy victim of old age, sorrow and death,

more transient than a dew drop on a blade of grass, nothing more or less than the product of the five elements.

This antagonistic attitude toward embodiment is still partly present in the *Yoga-Vasishtha* (VI.6.8), a tenth-century work that gestured toward a more integral teaching:

> Whatever happens to this insentient, nescient, vain, ungrateful and destructive bodily "stone"—that it deserves well.

Alongside statements of this kind, however, we also find refreshingly positive affirmations in this splendid scripture of nondualist Yoga. For instance, in one passage (IV.23.18) the body is said to be a source of sorrow and pain only for the spiritually blind, whereas it is a wellspring of unimaginable bliss for the sages. As the composer of the *Yoga-Vasishtha* puts it:

> This [body] is intended for his [i.e., the yogin's] enjoyment and liberation. It resembles a sage's grove. One's own body, [which is like] a big city, is for [the experience of] bliss, not suffering. (IV.23.2)

> As an accomplished charioteer guides the chariot with dexterity, so must this body likewise not be treated thoughtlessly. (IV.10.44)

> The wholesome (*sat*) body is destroyed in an instant by the mind that produces unwholesome (*asat*) volitions, rather like a baked [clay] doll [is broken] by a child. (IV.10.45)

The influence of Tantrism on the author of the *Yoga-Vasishtha* is quite obvious. For in the most progressive Tantras the body is celebrated as the abode of the Goddess or the temple of the Divine. This same view is captured in the *Yoga-Shikha-Upanishad* (V.4b), which states:

> The body is said to be the dwelling-place of Vishnu, bestowing perfection on all embodied [beings].

Here the body is no longer regarded as being merely a despicable aggregate of vile substances, nor as a pain-inflicting and impure envelope that conceals one's true essence. Rather, it is consecrated as the effluence and vessel of the ultimate Reality without which the individual would never see the dawn of enlightenment. This Tantric reappraisal of the body was fully elaborated and concretized in Hatha-Yoga.

THE FORCEFUL YOGA OF IMMORTALITY

The word *hatha* means simply "force." Thus, Hatha-Yoga is the forceful approach to liberation. However, the Sanskrit scriptures also furnish an esoteric explanation according to which the syllable *ha* stands for the sun and *tha* for the moon. Of course, these are not the luminaries of the physical firmament but inner realities, the positive and the negative psychosomatic current. Hatha-Yoga is said to consist in the deliberate merging (yoga) of these two psychospiritual principles, which yields the bliss of ecstasy.

The origin of Hatha-Yoga is still obscure. This tradition probably emerged in the eighth or ninth centuries A.D., as the final phase of the widely diffused siddha cult. The siddhas were accomplished masters who had not only realized the Divine but also acquired an assortment of paranormal powers (siddhi), which made them Godlike hierophants. In their circles, the "cultivation of the body" played a central role.

The founder of this physical Yoga is supposed to be the legendary Gorakshanatha (in Hindi: Gorakhnath), who is traditionally credited with the authorship of the two oldest but no longer extant treatises on Hatha-Yoga. His teacher, Matsyendra (c. 950 A.D.), is remembered as the author of such works as the *Kaula-Jnana-Nirnaya*. Though this work was probably composed no earlier than the eleventh century A.D., it contains authentic teachings of Matsyendra's school, known as Kaula.

This scripture is filled with all kinds of esoteric lore. Matsyendra's basic philosophy is clearly nondualist, and the practical path of realization outlined in the *Nirnaya* combines the striving for liberation with magical goals, as is typical of the Tantras. The teachings are a mixture of Goddess worship, complex yogic visualization, and physical manipulations such as postures and locks, as well as ritual sexuality.

In contrast to Matsyendra's left-hand teachings, Gorakshnatha preached a celibate, more ascetic approach. However, in his school we also find a curious combination of lofty ideals and magical concerns. Because of this, some scholars have seen in Hatha-Yoga merely a symptom of spiritual decline. For instance, the German Indologist J.W. Hauer characterized this branch of Yoga as

> a typical product of the period of decline of the Indian mind, which in spite of all assurances to the opposite is far from the ruthlessly honest urge towards a full clarification, the liberation of the soul and the experience of the ultimate reality. . . . Hathayoga has a strong touch of a coarse method of suggestion and is intimately linked with magic and sexuality.[1]

This harsh judgement is not entirely unfounded. Too often, practitioners of this branch of Yoga have lost sight of the high spiritual ideals of the great masters. We must not judge a movement by the failures of those who missed the mark, however, but by the mark itself. In that light, we cannot possibly find fault with the basic intent of Hatha-Yoga, which is to include the body in the process of spiritual transformation.

As much as any other type of Yoga, Hatha-Yoga purports to be a path to liberation. According to the classical manuals, it is meant to serve as a ladder to the spiritual heights of Raja-Yoga. The author of the *Hatha-Yoga-Pradipika* (IV.102) expressly declares:

> All the means of Hatha[-Yoga] are for [reaching] perfection in Raja-Yoga. A person who is rooted in Raja-Yoga conquers death.

Hatha-Yoga has undoubtedly contributed much that is essential and valuable, and to see in it merely a gross denigration of the lofty ideals of India's spirituality is unwarranted and inexcusable. It is an authentic continuation of the experimental and candid approach of Tantrism.

According to Tantrism, the body is an instrument of liberation, and illness or premature death are seen as severe handicaps on the spiritual path. Hence Hatha-Yoga aims in all its techniques at steeling the physical body so that eventually, upon the dawning of enlightenment, it can bear the diamond hardness of the ultimate Being. As the *Gheranda-Samhita* (I.8) declares:

Like an unbaked urn left in water, the [bodily] vessel is ever
[so soon] decayed. Baked well in the fire of Yoga the vessel becomes purified [and enduring].[2]

The *hatha-yogins* strive after liberation in a perfected body
(*siddha-deha*) that is free from illness and weakness and without the
limitations forming part of the ordinary mortal body. In the *Yoga-
Bija*, a short Sanskrit tract, two kinds of body are distinguished:
that which is "cooked," or matured, and that which is "uncooked."

The former body has been hardened in the fire of Yoga and
hence is also called *yoga-deha*. The *Yoga-Vasishtha* refers to it as the
ativahika, or superconductive body.[3] In accordance with the
nondualist philosophy of this work, the visible human body is a
mere illusion, and in reality there is only the omnipotent spiritual
body.[4] The *Yoga-Shikha-Upanishad* (I.40–42), again, contains the following pertinent verses:

Gradually withdrawing from the great elements and their po-
tentials (tanmatra), the body composed of the seven humors is
progressively consumed by the fire of Yoga.

That fire is not merely a metaphor but a hidden reference to an
actual psychoalchemical process triggered by the awakening of the
serpent power (kundalini), as will be explained shortly. The *Upanishad* next states that even the Gods cannot perceive this yogic body,
which is exempt from modification and bondage and possesses
various magical powers. Then we read:

The body [of the yogin] is like the ether, even purer than the
ether and is seen to be subtler than the subtle, coarse and yet
not coarse, insentient and yet sentient. (I.42)

This is the Body of the Divine itself. According to the *Siddha-
Siddhanta-Paddhati*, ascribed to Gorakshanatha, there is no existence without embodiment. The text distinguishes six kinds of
bodies (*pinda*), corresponding to levels of embodiment:

1. *para-pinda*   — transcendental body
2. *anadi-pinda*   — beginningless body,
                         prior to cosmic manifestation

3. *adya-pinda*	— original body, the first level of cosmic existence, corresponding to the "golden germ" (*hiranya-garbha*) in Vedanta
4. *mahasakara-pinda*	— cosmic body, the collective existence of higher levels of reality
5. *prakriti-pinda*	— natural body, produced by the conjunction of male and female principles, comprising also the psychomental faculties
6. *garbha-pinda*	— womb-born body, the flesh-and-blood vehicle

The *para-pinda* is the all-comprising Body of the Absolute, Shiva, which consists of pure Awareness. The other five bodies are progressively coarser manifestations of that universal Body. The uterine body is our familiar physical vehicle composed of the five material elements recognized in Indian cosmology.

For karmic reasons, we identify with the lowest manifestation of the Divine, which is our physical body. The cathartic processes of Hatha-Yoga aim at correcting this tunnel vision and restoring us to the glory of the highest Body, which is immortal. Some schools of Hatha-Yoga pursue physical immortality, but this is a sheer impossibility. The material realm is subject to change and final decay. Even the subtle levels of manifestation are exempt from entropy. After many billions of years the universe as a whole is destined to vanish.

Only the Divine itself is immune to the ravages of time. Those who have awakened in or as the Divine alone escape mortality. These liberated beings may, as divine incarnations (avatara), volunteer to assume a subtle body or even to be embodied on the material plane, but in that case they too cannot change the final destiny of all manifest things. At the appointed time, their body-mind will die, and they will simply be present again as pure Being-Awareness—the same universal Reality from which they were not distinct before or during their brief spell of embodiment.

AWAKENING THE SERPENT POWER

Hatha-Yoga, like most Tantric schools, operates on the basis of what has been called "esoteric anatomy." Acknowledging the seniority of Consciousness and of the subtle, psychospiritual structures over the physical dimension, the Tantric adepts focused on working directly with the human mind and energy field (the "subtle body").

The principal organs of the subtle body are the psychospiritual centers (cakra), the network of channels (nadi) carrying the life force (prana), and the most potent kundalini force, which is considered as the true dynamo of the spiritual process.

The main contribution of Hatha-Yoga lies in its innovative series of purification practices intended to remove blockages in the subtle channels. The masters of this branch of Yoga have also greatly elaborated the physical exercises, such as the postures (asana), seals (mudra), and locks (bandha), as well as the breathing techniques.

The purpose of all these practices is to interrupt the cyclic flow of the life force in the body and to concentrate it along the bodily axis, in the central channel known as sushumna-nadi. This laserlike focusing of the vital energy is thought to awaken the mysterious serpent force, or kundalini-shakti, about which the Hatha-Yoga-Pradipika (III.107) says that "he who knows her knows Yoga."

Ordinarily, the kundalini rests latent or coiled up at the lowest psychospiritual center, corresponding to the nerve plexus at the end of the spinal column. The kundalini is stirred into action by the psychosomatic heat generated when the life force enters the central channel. It then stretches upward toward the center at the crown of the head. This process, which is at the core of the Tantric path, is called sat-cakra-bheda, or "piercing of the six centers."

The kundalini is comparable to a vast reservoir of energy available to those who possess the key to it. Not only does it bestow on the adepts all the magical powers imaginable, but it also enables them to transcend space-time. The Hatha-Yoga-Pradipika states:

> The yogin who stirs up the [serpent] power enjoys perfection (siddhi). What more need be said? He playfully conquers time. (III.120)

The conquest of time is victory over death. In Sanskrit the word *kala* means both "time" and "death." To transcend space-time is to win immortality, for the transcendental Reality is eternal. The kundalini process is introduced as the means whereby this great feat can be accomplished.

> Sun and Moon establish time in the form of day and night. The *sushumna* is the consumer of time. This is said to be a [great] secret. (IV.17)

It is clear from the last sentence that this stanza is to be understood not literally but symbolically. "Sun" and "Moon" are the left and right channels that wind around the central channel in helical fashion. So long as the life force circulates through them, the human body-mind is moved through the ordinary ebb and flow of consciousness. However, mind and time stand still when the life current enters the axial channel. Then there is only the bliss of Reality. This is spelled out in the above-quoted text as follows:

> Where the mind is absorbed there the life force (*pavana*) is suspended; and where the life force is suspended, there the mind is absorbed. (IV.23)

> Both mind and life force are mingled like milk and water, and the activities of mind and life force concur. Where the life force [is active], there is mental activity; where the mind [is active], there is activity of the life force. (IV.24)

> Upon the stilling of the one, the other is stilled [as well]. When one is active, the other [too] is active. When both are in motion, the host of senses are active. When both are stationary, the state of liberation is attained. (IV.25)

The aroused kundalini extends itself, like a rearing cobra, toward the crown center. In order to reach that spot, which is pictured as Shiva's mountain seat, the serpent power must traverse the six major psychospiritual centers strung along the bodily axis as pearls on a string.

In ascending order, the six cakras are the *mula-adhara* ("root-base"), *svadhishthana* ("own-place"), *mani-pura* ("jeweled city"), *anahata* ("unstruck"), *vishuddha* ("pure"), and *ajna* ("command").

These six centers are thought of as the limbs composing the luminous body of the kundalini. They are also frequently referred to as lotuses that open up as the serpent power ascends.

The final station of the kundalini is the *sahasrara* center, depicted as a thousand-petaled lotus. There the dynamic force, which is an aspect of the divine Shakti, reunites with the static transcendental power, or Shiva. At first this blissful union is very brief, but through unfaltering effort it can gradually be prolonged.

This profound ecstatic experience is supposed to differ essentially from its equivalent in non-Tantric schools. Sir John Woodroffe, without whose pioneering work the Yoga of the Tantras would still be a sealed book, tackled this important issue head on.[5] He observed that followers of the non-Tantric paths of meditation tend to ignore the fact that body and mind are in constant interaction. They typically neglect the body or undermine their health by engaging in all manner of self-mortification, which is apt to produce psychotic states rather than genuine spiritual realizations.

Thus, noted Woodroffe, it is possible to be successful in meditation and yet be physically weak and sick. The non-Tantric adepts, though capable of all kinds of psychic feats, are seldom concerned with the fate of their body. Consequently, they are also not able to determine the moment of their death. In Hatha-Yoga, by contrast, conscious dying at the moment of one's own choosing is a vitally important practice.

Above all, the enlightenment of the non-Tantric adepts is said to lack the realization of bodily bliss. The ecstasy of the non-Tantrics does not include the desired kundalini awakening. Their experience of bliss is therefore entirely transcendental and exclusive of the bodily dimension. However, the hatha-yogins aspire to bring down that bliss into the human frame.

The arousing of the latent force within the body and its controlled guidance upward through the six centers is claimed to lead to a more complete enlightenment than is the case with ordinary spiritual methods. The Tantric adepts gain both liberation (*mukti*) and world enjoyment (*bhukti*) in the deepest sense.

Tantric spirituality seeks to bring the Divine down into the very cells of the body. The Tantras affirm again and again that the body is the Goddess. In enlightenment, when the entire body is filled with radiance, that fundamental Tantric axiom is experientially validated. The physical body is experienced as an unbounded vibrating force field that is connected with all beings and things.

Clearly, the new way of Tantrism and Hatha-Yoga created unique opportunities, but it also conjured up new dangers. The scriptures unanimously warn about the possible risks of awakening the serpent power. The kundalini is stated to lead sages to freedom but fools into more profound bondage. Just how great those risks can be we learn from the staggering kundalini experience of Gopi Krishna, who made this phenomenon known to large circles in the West:

> There was a sound like a nerve thread snapping and instantaneously a silvery streak passed zigzag through the spinal cord, exactly like the sinuous movement of a white serpent in rapid flight, pouring an effulgent, cascading shower of brilliant vital energy into my brain, filling my head with a blissful lustre in place of the flame that had been tormenting me for the last three hours. Completely taken by surprise at this sudden transformation of the fiery current, darting across the entire network of my nerves only a moment before, and overjoyed at the cessation of pain, I remained absolutely quiet and motionless for some time, tasting the bliss of relief with a mind flooded with emotion, unable to believe I was really free of the horror.[6]

As it turned out, Krishna had not yet passed through the crisis. The kundalini reared its head again and again over many years, causing him considerable physical discomfort and mental distress. At times he thought he would die, at other times he feared for his sanity. His case is not unique either.[7] However, once the awakened kundalini had stabilized, he found himself in a different world. As he explained:

> I do not claim that I see God, but I am conscious of a Living Radiance both within and outside of myself. In other words, I have gained a new power of perception, not present before. The luminosity does not end with my waking time. It

persists even in my dreams. In every state of being—eating, drinking, talking, working, laughing, grieving, walking, or sleeping—I always dwell in a rapturous world of light.[8]

Gopi Krishna freely admitted to possessing none of the magical powers traditionally thought to be associated with a fully active kundalini. However, his inner environment had been radically altered, and this included heightened creativity and certain psychic abilities. He felt his years of tribulation had been well worth it.

While Krishna's intriguing experience supports some of the traditional claims, it cannot be said to be entirely typical. For his kundalini awakening occurred spontaneously and without the guidance of a qualified teacher.

It is possible that it did not represent a full awakening in the traditional sense. However, Krishna's description of his experience contains sufficient information to encourage further study of this phenomenon.

It is possible that kundalini awakenings were known already in pre-Tantric times, but we have no evidence suggesting that their full significance had been realized at that time. This was possible only within the framework of Tantrism, which entailed a general reappraisal of the physical realm and the human body.

Gopi Krishna contends that every mystical experience, and in fact all creativity, is due to kundalini activity.[9] However, this claim makes sense only inasmuch as the kundalini could be said to be the connecting link between the physical and the spiritual dimension within each individual. But clearly there are physical and mental symptoms associated with the aroused kundalini that allow us to distinguish between the kundalini as a metaphysical force and the kundalini as an experiential phenomenon. The latter has been dubbed "physio-kundalini" by the American psychiatrist Lee Sannella.[10]

Evidently, not all creative work and all mystical experiences involve the dramatic psychosomatic manifestations that are reported of actual kundalini awakenings. Tantrism and Hatha-Yoga have devised methods by which such awakenings can be brought about under controlled conditions. This is precisely the paramount significance of these two traditions.

With the innovative teachings of Tantrism and Hatha-Yoga, India's spirituality reached a point where it was ready for the great encounter with the West. Alas, at that time, the Western world was still quite unprepared for an ecumenical dialogue. In fact, it is really only today, after centuries of Christian dualism and body-negativity followed by scientific materialism, that Western thinking has arrived at an auspicious juncture where we are able to critically assess our own heritage and the legacy of the East.

Above all, we have begun to understand something of the spiritual significance of the body. This turning point is epitomized in the work of Alexander Lowen, F.M. Alexander, Ashley Montagu, Moshe Feldenkrais, Stanley Keleman, Ida Rolf, Ken Dychtwald, Deane Juhan, and others.[11] This promising new trend has found a most articulate spokesman in the Canadian historian Morris Berman. He wrote:

> Modern science and technology are based not only on a hostile attitude toward the environment, but on the repression of the body and the unconscious; and unless these can be recovered, unless participating consciousness can be restored in a way that is scientifically (or at least rationally) credible and not merely a relapse into naive animism, then what it means to be a human being will forever be lost.[12]

In our postmodern attempt to recover the body as a living reality, we need not start from scratch. The Eastern traditions contain invaluable insights, empirical evidence, and several full-fledged psychotechnologies that can help us greatly in our own quest for self-understanding.

NOTES

1. J.W. Hauer, *Der Yoga: Ein indischer Weg zum Selbst* (Stuttgart: Kohlhammer Verlag, 1958), p. 271.

2. Remarkably enough, this view was anticipated by the ancient *Chandogya-Upanishad* (VIII.12.1), which contains the statement that "This [body] is the abode of the immortal, bodiless Self." However, the time was

not yet ripe for this insight to be translated into a more complete body-positive philosophy and practice. The overall orientation of this *Upanishad* is still ascetical.

3. The term *ativahika* is composed of *ati* ("extremely") and the root *vah* ("to carry").

4. See, for instance, *Yoga-Vasishtha* III.57.296. According to III.332, however, both the physical and the spiritual body are inexistent and pure apparitions of the One Being.

5. See A. Avalon [alias Sir J. Woodroffe], *The Serpent Power* (New York: Dover Publications, 1974), pp. 289ff. The first edition of this work was published in 1919.

6. Gopi Krishna, *Kundalini: Evolutionary Energy in Man* (London: Robinson & Watkins, 1971), p. 66.

7. See, for instance, the description by B.S. Goel, *Third Eye and Kundalini* (Kurukshetra: Third Eye Foundation of India, 1986).

8. G. Krishna, *The Real Nature of Mystical Experience* (New Delhi: Kundalini Research and Publication Trust, 1979), p. 28.

9. See G. Krishna, *Kundalini: The Secret of Yoga* (New Delhi: Kundalini Research and Publication Trust, 1978), pp. 180ff.

10. See L. Sannella, *The Kundalini Experience: Psychosis or Transcendence?* (Lower Lake, CA: Integral Publishing, 1987).

11. See A. Lowen, *The Language of the Body* (New York: Collier Books, 1971) and *Bioenergetics* (New York: Coward, McCann & Geoghegan, 1975); F.M. Alexander, *The Resurrection of the Body* (New York: Dell Publishing, 1971); A. Montagu, *Touching: The Human Significance of the Skin* (New York: Harper & Row, 1971); M. Feldenkrais, *Awareness through Movement* (New York: Harper & Row, 1972); S. Keleman, *Your Body Speaks Its Mind: The Bio-Energetic Way to Greater Emotional and Sexual Satisfaction* (New York: Simon & Schuster, 1975); I. Rolf, *Rolfing: The Integration of Human Structures* (Santa Monica, CA: Dennis-Landman, 1977); K. Dychtwald, *Bodymind* (Los Angeles: J.P. Tarcher, 1986); D. Juhan, *Job's Body: A Handbook for Bodywork* (Barrytown, NY: Station Hill Press, 1987).

12. M. Berman, *The Reenchantment of the World* (New York: Bantam Books, 1984), p. 125. See also his *Coming to Our Senses: Body and Spirit in the Hidden History of the World* (New York: Simon & Schuster, 1989).

EPILOGUE

MYTHIC AND INTEGRAL SPIRITUALITY

The most obvious result of the foregoing inquiry is that India's spiritual heritage cannot be subsumed under such headings as "flight from reality," "rigid asceticism," "antisocial transcendentalism," and so on. Rather, as we have seen, the immensely versatile spirituality of the Indian subcontinent comprises two broad tendencies that are markedly distinct.

The one tendency is expressive of the magic-mythic structure of consciousness, while the other tendency embodies a vital urge toward synthesis and integration, which has asserted itself consistently and with increasing force in the long spiritual evolution of the Indian branch of the human family.

Mythic and holistic spirituality not only differ in their theoretical presuppositions—their metaphysical and ethical points of departure—but they are also dissimilar in the structure of their proposed paths and their conception of the ultimate goal of spiritual life.

When we study India's sacred scriptures, we can witness an unmistakable progression in the inclusiveness of approach. Natural as this may appear, it is a fact of no mean significance and one which can only be fully appreciated on the basis of psychohistory, as outlined in chapter 1. For this progression cannot be explained merely in terms of an inevitable and normal elaboration of the technical and theoretical aspects of spirituality. Instead, we must recognize it as being primarily an advancement to ever more integral insights and attitudes, rooted in subtle but profound changes within consciousness itself.

The truth of this can best be seen when we compare the spiritual traditions at the two extreme ends of this protracted development, which covers more than four thousand years. On one end are the magic-mythic teachings of the Vedas and early *Upanishads*, and on the other end are the holistic schools of later Hinduism and Buddhism. The former represent as it were an amplified version of the archaic *participation mystique*, whereas the latter are of the nature of a mystical experimentalism that is consolidated by rational thought. In between, we have the early teaching of the *Bhagavad-Gita*, which gestures toward a more integral view of life, though still limited by the hierarchic social system of Brahmanism.

Later integral teachings often tend to be more obviously critical of the Hindu caste system and also far more tolerant toward the hidden outcastes—women. Another conspicuous indicator of the holistic type of spirituality is the unlimited range of means and devices that are employed to achieve the transmutation of consciousness. In fact, in such pronouncedly experimental traditions as Tantrism, anything can be turned into a spiritual trigger: social interaction, ritual, bodily disciplines, emptying of the mind, visualization, sexuality, or love-devotion (bhakti).

Amazingly enough, even the violent emotion of hate is thought to be a suitable vehicle for channeling energy and attention to accomplish spiritual ends. Thus, the *Bhagavata-Purana* (III.16.31), which is India's most substantial and eloquent work on the Yoga of devotion, also knows of a Yoga of hatred (*samrambha-yoga*). The idea and theoretical justification behind this approach is stated to be this:

> All human emotions are grounded in the erroneous conception of "I" and "mine." The Absolute, the universal Self, has neither "I"-sense nor emotions.

> Hence one should unite [with It] through friendship or enmity, peaceableness or fear, attachment or love. [The Absolute] sees no distinction whatsoever.[1]

A similar liberal orientation is also favored in the venerable *Vishnu-Purana*, a Sanskrit work dating back perhaps to the third century A.D. Here Shishupala, the king of the Cedis, is recorded as having won liberation through his extreme hatred of God Vishnu in three successive existences (as Hiranyakashipu, Ravana, and

Shishupala). Shishupala's Yoga of hatred was an unconscious spiritual discipline, but both these Puranas imply that it would be possible to adopt this course of negative emotion deliberately as well. However, this recommendation seems farfetched, and it certainly contradicts the wisdom of all other traditions, according to which evil intentions breed negative karma and unfavorable conditions of existence.

Even teachings of a more holistic bent express the need to stand free of negative emotions. They are neither to be suppressed nor to be actively invited. Wise practitioners simply witness hate, anger, fear, and all the other undesirable states when they happen to arise within their heart, without reacting to them. In due course, they will cease to be troublesome, because the ground in which they arise has been transformed.

Cultivation of the witness consciousness, called *sakshin* in Sanskrit, is the means of such psychic transformation. Mircea Eliade spoke of the witness consciousness as one of India's greatest discoveries.[2] He also called for a dialogue that transcends the barriers erected by philosophical jargon. Alas, for the adepts of India, the witness consciousness, or Spirit, is not a mere abstract concept but a living reality. Eliade did not tell us how we can overcome the handicap of language without delving into firsthand experience. In fact, he was quite reluctant to recommend Western students of India's cultural heritage to take up one or another spiritual path, putting his faith instead in thorough research.

But such intellectual study can disclose only so much before we encounter the walls of our own belief system. It seems impossible to truly understand India's gnostic teachings without some experience of the meditative state, which is the master key to the higher or subtle realities described in the sacred scriptures around the world. In the absence of personal experience, we can be sympathetic toward those traditions but still lack genuine understanding.

Only when we have had our own ingrained materialistic epistemology (or way of knowing) changed by firsthand spiritual experience can we fully understand the spiritual epistemology that informs the metaphysics of the world's sacred traditions. In his introduction to the anthology *Hindu Spirituality: Vedas through*

Vedanta, Krishna Sivaraman made this pertinent comment:

Tradition is not something that stands like a mountain for exploration. It functions rather as an archetype in relation to spirituality so that the approach that is proper to it must be one of evoking it by an attitude of respect and "receiving," of appropriation and advance.[3]

Respectful receptivity is not a disposition that is encouraged in our Western education system. If anything, that system fosters intellectual rapaciousness and arrogant rejection of transmitted ideas and values. Hence in dealing with sacred lore there is a crying need for balancing our inherited "scientific objectivism." Meditation can provide that counterweight.

IN DIALOGUE WITH INDIA

India's spirituality deserves a careful study, and one that is conducted not merely from an intellectual viewpoint. We cannot possibly be satisfied with the kind of summary dismissal exemplified by Arthur Koestler's following remark:

Mankind is facing its most deadly predicament since it climbed down from the trees; but one is reluctantly brought to the conclusion that neither Yoga, Zen, nor any other Asian form of mysticism has any significant advice to offer.[4]

Other critics are still more outspoken, suggesting that India's spiritual paths are fallacious and futile. The implication that they are the result of many centuries of self-deception, involving millions of people and several cultures, is simply preposterous. If any self-deception is involved, it is surely on the part of those critics who are unwilling to recognize the authenticity of the witness consciousness or mystical realization.

To dismiss India's spiritual heritage is to eliminate an essential aspect of human life and to effectively bar the way to a solution to our modern predicament. For it is becoming ever more patent that the contemporary crisis does not concern merely politics, economics, demographics, ecology, ideology, or morality, but affects all dimensions of contemporary humanity. Hence it calls for a complete reorientation of our core values and, in particular, our relationship to the all-comprising Reality in which we have our being.

Are we then to drop our secular lifestyle and convert to one or another sacred tradition that holds appeal for us? Some individuals have indeed tried to follow this route, though seldom with much success. Usually their lives are not any more authentic. They may read the Bible or the Upanishads regularly, pray and count beads or meditate and chant mantras, but they have not radically changed within themselves. Their narcissism has simply been transferred from the secular to the religious domain.

The depth of the psyche has not been converted, and they have remained spiritual dilettantes. Whereas in the past they were looking for personal fulfillment by climbing the corporate ladder and hoarding material goods, now they hope to find it through religious rituals and meanings. Most of these seekers are still out of touch with the larger Reality and, if anything, are more confused and unhappy, though it would take much insight and personal strength to admit this.

At any rate, while individuals may engage in such experiments, it is clear that as a civilization we cannot turn the clock back. We cannot adopt sacred traditions as we don a new fashionable garment. Most Westerners have become so estranged from their religious roots that they can no longer relate to Christianity or Judaism rightly. As a consequence, born-again Christians or Jews or converts to other religions tend to become fundamentalists, driven by a terrible need to believe in something.

Religious revivalism is not the answer to our present-day dilemma. Even though it is true that modern humanity must recover contact with the sacred Ground of existence, we will never succeed, individually or collectively, so long as our quest for spiritual wholeness is prompted by neurotic motivations of personal safety and belonging. But it would appear that self-alienation and Reality-alienation have progressed too far to be cured by an act of blind faith. Many converts to Yoga, Vedanta, Buddhism, Zen, Sufism, or native American or African worldviews project parental status upon these traditions and their authority figures, and in this way they seek to avoid personal responsibility.

Undoubtedly, participation in these traditions can give people a sense of identity, belonging, and security. It can even enhance a person's self-understanding to the point where a genuine approach to spirituality becomes possible. Yet, arguably, most men and women would derive as much benefit from some of the more down-to-earth Western approaches of self-discovery, such as bodywork or gestalt therapy.

It is easy to conceal one's psychological troubles under a smokescreen of religious enthusiasm, mechanical repetition of mantras, wholesale acceptance of a ready-made philosophy of life, passive waiting for the flash of enlightenment, or willing abandonment to any of the many saviors from the East or West. How can one possibly expect to actualize transcendental Being-Awareness when not even one's everyday awareness is functioning properly?

Converts to Eastern traditions face the added challenge of archaic beliefs and symbols that may excite the intellect and stimulate the imagination but are essentially alien to the modern psyche. Jean Gebser mentioned the interesting and typical example of a long-standing European devotee of Ramana Maharshi who, despite serious dedication and intensive meditation in apparently ideal surroundings, had failed to achieve the much-desired ecstatic experience. Gebser asked the decisive question:

> If fifteen years' instruction of a ready pupil by a unique master only produces this result, how about those adherents of Yoga in the United States and Europe who are mostly initiated into the secrets and rigors of Yoga by third or fourth hand?[5]

The sacred traditions are all initiatory by nature. The gnostic knowledge is transmitted from teacher to disciple, and it matters very much who the initiator is. One of the most common traps in spiritual life is to feel the call to teach long before one is ready. Impatient Western students have been known to assume the mantle of the teacher shortly after receiving their own preliminary initiation in the sacred mysteries. They have of course failed the very first test in spiritual life. This is unfortunate for them personally, but it is even more unfortunate and disadvantageous for those who have been initiated by such misguided teachers and impostors. For, according to tradition, initiations offered by unqualified teachers amount to very little.

The reason for this is that initiation is not about any communication of knowledge but involves rather the transmission of spiritual grace. It is a form of spiritual empowerment, and that empowerment can be only as genuine as the teacher who bestows it upon the disciple.

Eastern spiritual traditions have been abroad in Western countries for many decades, and one cannot help but wonder how few of the teaching lineages are truly empowered. But even when people are fortunate enough to come into contact with an authentically taught tradition, they still have to find the right response within themselves or the empowerment will fail to take root in them.

John Blofeld, a convert to Buddhism who had been fortunate enough to obtain proper initiation into the Vajrayana tradition, is a characteristic case in point. At the end of his commendable spiritual autobiography, he confessed with admirable honesty:

> Back in Bangkok amid the clamorous surroundings of a worldly city, with few friends to share my enthusiasm or to drive me forward with stern words of encouragement and by high example, the great urge which lay upon me daily in the mountains has sadly declined. No longer am I blessedly tormented by the Great Thirst; no longer do I maintain iron control over the sinews of body and spirit. I long to press forward along the Path, but not until I came to write this book did the longing revive sufficiently for me to renew my daily efforts, relinquished about a year ago. The future is still in my own hands; the longing to make good use of the fast-flying years is there; but whether I shall gather strength to press the great assault, steeling the will to gain all or perish—time alone will show.[6]

Blofeld's case is rare only in its self-honesty, but otherwise it is perfectly symptomatic of the enormous struggle and final failure experienced by many disillusioned Westerners who have

converted to an Eastern way of life. Forsaking their own cultural
roots, they also fail to assimilate the spirituality of the adopted culture, and thus only exacerbate their predicament. In another book,
Blofeld made this parallel admission:

> My own experience and that of a number of Zen followers
> among my Chinese and Western acquaintances incline me to
> think that, even after long years of effort, relatively few people
> using the direct approach manage to get beyond the elemen-
> tary stage of stilling the mind for a little while. Undoubtedly
> there are some who succeed in entering deep samadhi, reach-
> ing the state of bliss and going beyond that, but there would
> seem to be many more who do not. . . . I hasten to add
> that most of my successful Tantric friends are Mongols or
> Tibetans.[7]

In the early 1930s, Paul Brunton travelled to India in search of
truth and of himself, discovered Ramana Maharshi for the West,
and finally found the wisdom of the East and West within his own
psyche. Much later he commented:

> Those who are so fascinated by the ancient tenets and
> methods that they surrender themselves wholly to them are
> living in the past and are wasting precious time relearning
> lessons which they have already learned.[8]

Brunton went on to say that those who are drawn to the East
tend to be so predisposed by their own autosuggestion. They do
not understand that they were born in the West to learn particular
lessons there rather than in the Orient. He remarked about his own
earlier fascination with India's spiritual heritage that he was then
suffering from "Indolatry."[9] Next he candidly confessed:

> Because I was once responsible for turning a number of
> eyes towards India in search of light, I now feel morally re-
> sponsible for turning most of them back homewards again.
> This is not to be misunderstood, for it is not the same as asking
> people to ignore India. No! I say that we all should study and
> digest the Oriental wisdom. But I also say first, that we should
> not make it our sole and exclusive diet and second, that

we should cook, spice, and serve it in a form suitable to our Occidental taste.[10]

With Jean Gebser, we can understand the distinction between East and West as a difference in cognitive styles, or dominant structures of consciousness. The Eastern branch of the human family animates, for historical reasons, a type of mental consciousness that is still heavily steeped in the magical and mythic worldviews. By contrast, the Western hemisphere is largely ruled, to its own detriment, by the mental-rational consciousness.

It is evident from these psychohistorical considerations that, as distinct approaches to reality, East and West are unlikely ever to meet. Even when all the political iron curtains are lifted, a separative glass curtain remains. The metaphor of the glass curtain was introduced by the world-renowned historian Arnold Toynbee in a UNESCO radio discussion with philosopher Raghavan Iyer in 1959.[11] The two men concluded that the only way to deal with this semi-visible wall between East and West is to renounce all claims to uniqueness and to create a new humanism in whose vocabulary the word "foreigner" does not exist—an early expression of today's global philosophy.

Thus, even though East and West may not merge, it is possible for them to converge in a higher synthesis: the integral consciousness. In fact, such a convergence has become absolutely essential for the survival of the human family as a whole. What this involves on the individual level has been lucidly articulated by Jean Gebser:

> The new structure of consciousness has nothing to do with power, overpowering, or control. It can also not be aspired to but at best be elicited. Anyone who strives for it and thus endeavors to reach it mentally is from the outset doomed to failure. The same holds true of those who believe that mere wishing and the power of imagination—that is, mythically tinged volition—can bring about the actualization of the new mutation; and it is equally true of those who believe they can master this mutation by some machination, because this would only signal a relapse into magical compelling and being compelled.

What is needed is care, much patience, and the discarding of many preconceived opinions, wishful dreams, and blind demands; and it calls for a certain detachment toward oneself and the world, a gradually maturing balance between all inherent components and consciousness structures, in order that we may create a basis for the leap into the new mutation.[12]

This integral attitude may be fruitfully combined with certain practices, such as meditation or a suitably modified version of Hatha-Yoga. Yet these techniques are of secondary importance, and their only value lies in facilitating that inner attitude. Unless this is clearly understood, no amount of expertise in, or dedication to, any of the esoteric disciplines can be of real consequence and may even prove inimical to a person's maturation toward the integral consciousness.

In what way, and to what extent, Eastern methods and concepts can and should be utilized cannot be decided here. It seems obvious, however, that in most instances some form of meditative practice is called for in order to supplement and reinforce the cultivation of openness and lucidity.

The ultimate criterion for the justification and usefulness of any particular practice will have to be whether or not it results in liberation, understood not as an escape from the world but as transparency:

> The unfragmented, ego-free person who no longer sees parts but realizes the "Itself" (*Sich*) as the spiritual form of the being of man and world, apprehends the Whole, the diaphainon that "lies before" all origin and that shines through everything. For him there is neither heaven nor hell, neither this world nor the next, neither ego nor world, neither immanence nor transcendence. . . . He does not need to re-link (religion) with it, for it is "preligious": It is present in an achronic, atemporal way that corresponds to his ego-free being. . . . The timeless becomes time-free, voidness becomes fullness and in the diaphaneity the diaphainon, the Spiritual, becomes apprehensible: The origin is the present. We ware the Whole, and the Whole wares us.[13]

This mutual "waring" (*wahren*) is an actualization in which Reality, or the truth, is communicated and preserved. This is not intended as a description of yogic ecstasy (samadhi), or Zen satori, or any other peak experience in Maslow's sense, even though these may anticipate, and be directly or indirectly instrumental in achieving, the breakthrough to the realization of the Being/Becoming continuum that Jean Gebser had in mind when writing these words.

In India this living in diaphaneity is known as sahaja, the natural or spontaneous state, in which everything falls into its proper place. All blinds drop, and the blue hills are simply blue hills, the white clouds are simply white clouds. Nirvana equals samsara. This is no goal and even less an ultimate purpose or state. It is a process that is synchronous with the unfolding of life itself.

The difference between the sahaja state and conventional forms of ecstatic realization (samadhi) has been carefully delineated by the Western spiritual teacher Da Free John (Franklin Jones).[14] As he elaborated, the highest mystical condition of conventional spirituality is the transconceptual ecstasy (nirvikalpa-samadhi), which is based on the ascent of attention. In this state, attention is exclusively focused within the topmost psycho-spiritual center of the human body-mind, which he calls the "brain core."

This type of ecstasy involves a genuine merging with the transcendental Reality, but this realization is exclusive of the manifest dimension. By contrast, the sahaja or "natural" state is not accompanied by any fixation of attention. Rather the ebb and flow of attention itself is transcended. Whether the sahaja-yogins perceive external objects or contemplate the vast inner world, they do not merely witness all phenomena appearing in consciousness but, paradoxically, also *are* those phenomena.

As the integral consciousness is realized by a growing number of individuals, its harmonizing effect will spread in ever wider circles to all human cultures. This is not an altogether new vision, as we have seen in our discussion of the Hindu moral ideal of loka-samgraha or the Buddhist bodhisattva ideal. However, for the first time in human history, we are in a position to realize it on a truly global scale, apart from all ideological parochialism and ethno-centrism. This is a vision that seems worthy of our aspiration and effort, individually and collectively.

NOTES

1. *Bhagavata-Purana* VII.1.23ff.

2. See M. Eliade, *Yoga: Immortality and Freedom* (Princeton, NJ: Princeton University Press, 1970), p. xx.

3. K. Sivaraman, ed., *Hindu Spirituality: Vedas through Vedanta* (New York: Crossroad, 1989), p. xxviii.

4. A. Koestler, *The Lotus and the Robot* (London: Danube Books, 1966), p. 282.

5. J. Gebser, *Asien lächelt anders* [Asia Smiles Differently] (Berlin: Verlag Ullstein, 1968), p. 108. The English rendering is by the present author.

6. J. Blofeld, *The Wheel of Life* (London: Rider, 1972), p. 285.

7. J. Blofeld, *The Tantric Mysticism of Tibet: A Practical Guide* (New York: Dutton, 1970), p. 217.

8. P. Brunton, *The Orient: Its Legacy to the West* (Burdett, NY: Larson Publications, 1987), p. 15. This is volume 10 of *The Notebooks of Paul Brunton*.

9. *Ibid.*, p. 21.

10. *Ibid.*, pp. 27–28.

11. See, R. Iyer, ed., *The Glass Curtain Between Asia and Europe: A Symposium on the Historical Encounters and the Changing Attitudes of the Peoples of the East and the West* (London: Oxford University Press, 1965), pp. 329–349.

12. J. Gebser, *Ursprung und Gegenwart* (Stuttgart: Deutsche Verlags-Anstalt, 1966), I. p. 319. The English rendering is by the present author.

13. *Ibid.*, p. 559.

14. See Bubba [Da] Free John, *The Enlightenment of the Whole Body* (Middletown, CA: Dawn Horse Press, 1978). See also his *The Paradox of Instruction* (San Francisco: Dawn Horse Press, 1977), which contains much valuable discussion of the distinction between conventional samadhi and whole-body enlightenment.

SELECT BIBLIOGRAPHY

THIS BIBLIOGRAPHY includes only publications that the general reader will find useful. For further reading, the comprehensive bibliographies by Howard R. Jarrell (1981) and Robin Monro *et al.* (1989), as well as the bibliographies in the standard works on Yoga and Tantrism by Mircea Eliade (1970) and Agehananda Bharati (1965) may profitably be consulted.

Aurobindo [Ghose]. *The Life Divine.* Pondicherry: Sri Aurobindo Ashram, 1955. 2 vols.

———. *On Yoga.* Pondicherry: Sri Aurobindo Ashram, 1955.

Avalon, A. [alias Sir J. Woodroffe]. *The Serpent Power.* New York: Dover Books, 1974.

———. *Tantra of the Great Liberation.* New York: Dover Books, 1972.

Ayyangar, T.R.S., transl. *The Yoga Upanisads.* Adyar: Adyar Library, 1952.

Bharati, A. *The Tantric Tradition.* London: Rider, 1965.

Blofeld, J. *The Wheel of Life.* London: Rider, 1972.

———. *The Tantric Mysticism of Tibet.* New York: Dutton, 1970.

Brunton, Paul. *The Notebooks of Paul Brunton.* Burdett, NY: Larson Publications, 1984–1988. 16 vols.

Chauduri, H. and Spiegelberg, F., eds. *The Integral Philosophy of Sri Aurobindo.* London: Allen & Unwin, 1960.

Conze, E. *Buddhist Thought in India.* London: Allen & Unwin, 1962.

Conze, E. et al., eds., *Buddhist Texts through the Ages.* New York: Harper Torchbooks, 1962.

Eliade, M. *Yoga: Immortality and Freedom.* Princeton, NJ: Princeton University Press, 1970.

———. *Patanjali and Yoga.* New York: Schocken Books, 1969.

Evans-Wentz, W.Y. *Tibetan Yoga and Secret Doctrines.* London: Oxford University Press, 1935.

Feuerstein, G. *Yoga: The Technology of Ecstasy.* Los Angeles: J.P. Tarcher, 1989.

———. *Encyclopedic Dictionary of Yoga.* New York: Paragon House, 1990.

———. *Sacred Paths.* Burdett, NY: Larson Publications, 1991.

———. *Holy Madness: The Shock Tactics and Radical Teachings of Crazy-Wise Adepts, Holy Fools, and Rascal Gurus.* New York: Paragon House, 1991.

———. *The Yoga-Sutra of Patanjali: A New Translation and Commentary.* Rochester, VT: Inner Traditions, 1989.

———. *Introduction to the Bhagavad-Gita: Its Philosophy and Cultural Setting.* Wheaton, IL.: Quest Books, 1983.

Frawley, D. *Gods, Sages and Kings: Vedic Secrets of Ancient Civilization.* Salt Lake City, UT: Passage Press, 1991.

Gebser, J. *The Ever-Present Origin.* Athens: Ohio University Press, 1985.

Ghosh, S. *The Original Yoga as Expounded in Siva-Samhita, Gheranda-Samhita and Patanjala Yoga-Sutra.* New Delhi: Munshiram Manoharlal, 1980.

Gopi Krishna. *Kundalini: Evolutionary Energy in Man.* Boulder, CO: Shambhala Publications, 1971.

Govinda, A. *Foundations of Tibetan Mysticism.* London: Rider, 1972.

———. *The Way of the White Clouds.* London: Rider, 1972.

Grof, S., ed. *Ancient Wisdom and Modern Science.* New York: SUNY Press, 1984.

——— and C. Grof, *The Stormy Search for the Self: A Guide to Personal Growth through Transformational Crisis.* Los Angeles: J.P. Tarcher, 1990.

Heard, J. and Cranson, S.L., eds. *Reincarnation: An East-West Anthology.* New York: Crown, 1961.

Hill, W.D.P. *The Bhagavadgita.* London: Oxford University Press, 1953.

Hume, R.E. *The Thirteen Principal Upanishads.* London: Oxford University Press, 1931.

Jarrell, H.R. *International Yoga Bibliography, 1950 to 1980.* Metuchen, NJ:

Scarecrow Press, 1981.

Jung, C.G. *Psychology and the East*. Princeton, NJ: Princeton University Press, 1978.

Koestler, A. *The Lotus and the Robot*. London: Danube Books, 1966.

Laski, M. *Ecstasy: A Study of Some Secular and Religious Experiences*. Los Angeles: J.P. Tarcher, 1990.

Maslow, A.H. *The Farther Reaches of Human Nature*. Harmondsworth, England: Pelican Books, 1973.

Monro, Robin, *Yoga Research Bibliography: Scientific Studies on Yoga and Meditation*. Cambridge, England: Yoga Biomedical Trust, 1989.

Prem, S.K. *The Yoga of the Bhagavat Gita*. Baltimore, MD: Penguin Books, 1973.

Radhakrishnan, S. *The Bhagavadgita*. London: Allen & Unwin, 1948.

Sangharakshita, B. *The Three Jewels*. London: Rider, 1967.

Sannella, L. *The Kundalini Experience: Psychosis or Transcendence?* Lower Lake, CA: Integral Publishing, 1987.

Tart, C. *Transpersonal Psychologies*. New York: Harper & Row, 1975.

Thapar, R. *A History of India*. Harmondsworth, England: Pelican Books, 1972.

Tucci, G. *The Theory and Practice of the Mandala*. London: Rider, 1969.

Vaughan, F. *The Inward Arc: Healing and Wholeness in Psychotherapy and Spirituality*. Boston/London: New Science Library/Shambhala, 1985.

Walsh, R. and F. Vaughan, eds. *Beyond Ego: Transpersonal Dimensions in Psychology*. Los Angeles: J.P. Tarcher, 1980.

Watts, A.W. *Psychotheraphy East and West*. New York: Mentor Books, 1961.

Wilber, K. *The Spectrum of Consciousness*. Wheaton, IL: Theosophical Publishing House, 1980.

——, et al., eds. *Transformations of Consciousness: Conventional and Contemplative Perspectives on Development*. Boston/London: New Science Library/Shambhala, 1986.

Zimmer, H. *Myths and Symbols in Indian Art and Civilization*. New York: Harper Torchbooks, 1962.

INDEX

A

abhimana, 121
abhinivesha, 64
abhyasa, 44, 46
Absolute, 190, 195, 196, 233, 255.
    See also God
Acaranga-Sutra (quoted), 53
action, 213–216, 237
Adam, 78
adept
    karma of, 45, 60
    and powers, 176
    and time, 70
adharma, and dharma, 62
adhikara, 215
adi-purusha, 123
advaita, 242
Advaita Vedanta, 36, 180, 182, 205, 242,
    253. See also Vedanta
Advaya-Taraka-Upanishad, 158
adya-pinda, 271
Agastya, 110
Agni-Purana (quoted), 266
aham brahma asmi, 157, 256
ahamkara, 80, 121, 171, 217
ahimsa, 105, 106, 206. See also nonharming
ajna-cakra, 158, 273
akala, 70
akarman, 214
akasha, 179
Akhilananda, Swami, 165, 166
Alarka, 73
Alexander, F.M., 277
alienation, from Self, 172
Alvars, 222
Amara-Kosha, 138
Amitabha, 247
amrita, 41
Amrita-Bindu-Upanishad, 196n
anabhidroha, 106
anadi-pinda, 270
anahata-cakra, 273
ananda, 233
ananda-maya-kosha, 193
Ananta, 42, 132
ananta, 132
ananta-samapatti, 132
anatman, 36, 52
anatomy, esoteric, 272
Andal, 224, 225

anga, 99
anger, 110, 140, 143, 236
Anguttara-Nikaya, 241
animan, 179
anna, 193
anna-maya-kosha, 193
anrishamsya, 106
anu-vrata, 207
apana, 74, 136, 137
aparigraha, 105, 108
Appar, 225
apratishta-nirvana, 247
arahant, 198, 245, 246, 248
Aristotle, 27–28
Arjuna, 13, 44, 86, 87, 207, 212, 213
Arnold, E., 11
art, 203, 204
artha, 189
arurukshu, 218
Aryans, Vedic, 65n
asamprajnata-samadhi, 154, 169, 170, 172,
    180, 183, 209n
asana, 130, 131, 132, 272
Asanga, 248
asat, 267
ascent, mystical, 29
asceticism, 122–125
    and body, 266
    and devotionalism, 227
    and mythic consciousness, 75, 205, 279
    and nonharming, 207
    and sacrifice, 123
    and suffering, 57
    and women, 200
ashaya, 126
ashrama, 48, 206
Asita Devala, 208
asmita, 64, 171
asparsha-yoga, 243
aspirant, spiritual, 93, 218, 219, 263
asrava, 61
asteya, 105, 108
astikya, 118
astral projection, 179
asura, 66
Atharva-Veda, 136, 256
Atharva-Veda (quoted), 96
ativahika, 270, 278n
Atma-Bodha, 119-120, 196n
atman, 33, 61, 144
attachment, 64, 140, 214, 215, 280